TRAUMA & ABUSE HEALING

TRAUMA & ABUSE
HEALING

*The Guide to Using Ritual
and Ceremony to Delight in Life*

Heidi Henyon

NEW YORK

LONDON • NASHVILLE • MELBOURNE • VANCOUVER

Trauma and Abuse Healing

The Guide to Using Ritual and Ceremony to Delight in Life

Published in New York, New York, by Morgan James Publishing in partnership with Difference Press. Morgan James is a trademark of Morgan James, LLC. www.MorganJamesPublishing.com

ISBN 9781642798753 paperback
ISBN 9781642798760 eBook
ISBN 9781642798777 audiobook
Library of Congress Control Number: 2019916224

Cover Concept and Design by:
Rachel Lopez
www.r2cdesign.com

Editor:
Moriah Howell

Book Coaching:
The Author Incubator

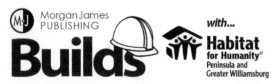

Morgan James is a proud partner of Habitat for Humanity Peninsula and Greater Williamsburg. Partners in building since 2006.

Get involved today! Visit
MorganJamesPublishing.com/giving-back

I want to dedicate this book to all those who are caught in the memories of abuse and trauma—may they find the inherent Joy and Wisdom that resides within and be Free—and to all those who have dedicated their lives to helping them.

Table of Contents

Chapter 1:   What I Want for My Clients 1

Chapter 2:   Stories of Healing .5

Chapter 3:   Why This Process. 13

Chapter 4:   How Does Ritual Work? 23

Chapter 5:   Finding Home 43

Chapter 6:   Releasing 63

Chapter 7:   Vision 81

Chapter 8:   Honoring Ourselves. 95

Chapter 9:   Obstacles You May Encounter 111

Chapter 10:   Conclusion 117

Ritual and Ceremony Check List. 121

Bibliography 123
Acknowledgments 125
About the Author 129
Thank You. 131

Chapter 1

What I Want
for My Clients

J. told me one day that she had been in therapy for years and was still traumatized every time the holiday season came around; she would be immobilized by the memories of her childhood sexual abuse for weeks. Sometimes, she was not even able to get out of bed.

How frustrating for her therapist to not be able to find the key to help J. unravel the trauma that had her stuck. It can be heart wrenching for you when your client is not moving through and is stuck in their trauma, caught in their fears.

Sometimes you just don't know what to do next. But that is what you do; you help others find the next step toward feeling whole, healed, or just simply safe to go about their daily lives. But it can sometimes seem to take a long time for your clients to have breakthroughs. When they look at you imploringly for answers and you're not sure what will help next, it can be frustrating for you.

J. changed to a therapist who was not as conventional as the last. This therapist had different tools, and in a few months, J. was so much better and was now coming off all of her meds with the help of her therapist.

It is also so rewarding and exciting when you see them have breakthroughs. Those ah-ha moments where pieces fall into place, their pain starts to dissipate just a little, and their confidence in their own healing grows.

What if you had another tool you could easily turn to that has helped thousands? What if you knew it was being used more and more every day by therapists, counselors, clergy, and many others to help their clients and that it had also gotten great results in prisons, group homes, and other community settings?

The tools I am talking about are ritual and ceremony. Ritual and ceremony have been used for centuries by indigenous groups to heal "an unrested soul." Rituals are part of our lives every day, but we do not tend to recognize them. We have very specific daily rituals. We tend to call them routines because we don't recognize the spiritual value of them.

For example, what is the first thing you do every morning? For many it is that cup of coffee, saying a prayer, or brushing our teeth. We repeat the same actions or at the very least very similar ones because they bring us comfort, help us to come back, and focus here where we are. What happens when you change the first rituals of your morning? Do you hear yourself saying to other people, "Oh, I'm a little off this morning—I broke my routine." Rituals that we repeat bring us comfort, a sense of peace, and grounding. Even when they are not the greatest for us, they still bring us comfort. They help us feel safe. They really are a spiritual act.

In rituals, the mind gets to relax and the subconscious feels safe. That is why so many can find comfort in the ritual of prayer and during journaling. These kinds of practices help our minds to calm by giving them something to focus on.

In this place of safety, we can explore our thoughts and memories in a more detached way or simply let go of them. Ritual also helps us touch those deeper places inside that truly do have the answers we need to take our next steps.

Ceremony is broadly defined as the celebration of an event. It can be spiritual in nature or not. When we join in rituals of a healing nature and ceremonies to celebrate what we have learned from the rituals with others to recognize us, our transformations become very powerful.

We are able to let go of fears, redefine our stories, and heal.

Many books have been written in great detail about meditation, ritual, and the mind—how the brain releases the "feel good" chemicals and how parts of the brain that we do not use regularly become active. Please see the bibliography for more detailed information. This book is a practical guide to start incorporating ceremony and ritual into your practice.

In these pages, you will learn a process that is easy, straightforward, and can be used for individual counseling as well as groups. It creates a community for your clients where they can feel safe to express themselves, learn to trust again, and have support from others.

Chapter 2

Stories of Healing

My Story

I always knew my childhood was rough, but I had no idea how rough. I had so few memories of that time until, at age fifty-four, they came flooding back.

I was on my normal Thursday visit with my dad. However, this time something didn't feel right. We were talking about mom's history, which is another crazy story for a different time, when I started to feel uneasy. Dad was saying he was sorry he left when we were young. He and Mom had been divorced for a while. Mom was stable and had a good man, who we called

Uncle Tom. She was going to marry him. Tom was a retired general and had a good reputation. Dad felt Tom loved Mom, my sister, and me. Tom seemed like a good man.

That bad feeling rose up again, and I tried to brush it away.

I left Dad's and was heading to my counselor's office. I will refer to her as M.B. I had known her for many years. She helped me when things got rough during my first marriage, and I was currently in that same place in my second.

By the time I got to her office, about half an hour later, I could barely function. I'm still not quite sure how I got in the door.

All I could see were flashes of hiding in a closet, being dragged out by my mother, and being told to shut up and do what I was told. After working with M.B. for a while, more memories surfaced. Things like my mother handing me to Uncle Tom. The details kept flooding in, and I didn't want to believe them. Sometimes, even today, I am surprised I made it through those months. I do know that my comfort and familiarity with ritual were critical to my quick recovery.

I won't get into the graphic detail, but let it suffice that I was sexually abused repeatedly from ages six to seven.

That first day and the next morning, I worked with M.B. intensely. She used a practice called Advanced Integrative Therapy (A.I.T.), and it truly saved me and helped me to get stable so I could make it home. For a short time after, I was simply in shock and full-blown P.T.S.D., but due to M.B.'s help and the rituals I knew, I was functional.

In between sessions with M.B., I used water rituals to help cleanse away my pain, earth rituals to stay grounded, and nature rituals to facilitate change. Some I had learned from Sobonfu Somé, my teacher from the Dagara tradition, some from other traditions I learned along the way, and some just seemed to come to me as I needed them.

M.B. also used rituals and ceremonies she learned during her studies to help me move through the pain and grief and get to a place of wholeness. I became fully-functioning in only a few months. Yes, a few months. I have had conversations with a number of therapists and friends who have dealt with issues of severe abuse like mine, and they are all surprised by how quickly I healed and was able to forgive those who allowed me to be hurt.

I believe I healed so quickly because of the transformational experience I had during rituals I participated in over the years prior, as well as the support I received from the community that I learned and shared these rituals with.

Consciously practicing ritual and ceremony changed the way I saw the world. They helped me to gain trust and confidence in myself to know there is something greater than my mind. I learned from being in the community of people also dedicated to healing that we all have our trials in life, and we can support each other through them and give back to one another.

I also believe that the rituals I learned and practiced prior to my memories returning prepared me for the day I had to face them. There is a strength that I see people gain, a way to be grounded and whole inside that comes from the practice of ritual.

Take my friend Shakti; she had been going through a lot. Her family was falling apart. The man she loved so dearly was lost in his own grief and panic, not knowing how to help his son. His son was lost in his own pain and in a terrible place. She was feeling alone and helpless.

I asked if she wanted to do a releasing ceremony with me.

She said, "Yes!" We spent a few hours by the pond on my property, pouring our hearts out to the water, the earth, and the sky. We asked for help and guidance for ourselves and our families. It was an intense let-go process. When it came to a natural close, we both felt a sense of hope and that something had lifted and shifted.

Less than a week later, Shakti told me that there had been a huge positive shift in her circumstance. The cycle that was perpetuating the grief and chaos was interrupted, allowing true healing to begin. Her son was getting the help he needed and began to stabilize. Her husband was released from the grips of his own panic and confusion and began to put the pieces of his life back together. Shakti began to feel she could breathe again in her own home. There was finally the space for healing to happen. A new day had dawned.

Ritual can be done one-on-one with clients and in community. I want to share a community story about ritual that really helped me heal quickly.

A few weeks before my memories came back, I had bought my ticket to go to California to help with a grief ritual my teacher Sobonfu Somé was facilitating. My friend Susan was hosting her. At this point, I had been studying the Dagara tradition for thirteen or fourteen years with Sobonfu. I thank God for this every day. It was the water rituals that I learned from Sobonfu that helped make it between visits to M.B.

When I went to California, I still was not able to talk openly about what I was going through. The shame and pain were too great. Susan and Sobonfu had no idea. They sensed something was going on but knew me well enough to understand that I would share when ready. When we started to build the shrines and preparing the space, I started to have those awful feelings again. I could barely talk and couldn't help with the preparations. I went to that place of being lost again and not present. P.T.S.D. had struck.

As soon as the space was opened, Susan took me to the shrine, but nothing would come out. I can't even remember if

I was crying. The next thing I knew, Susan was next to me and she was saying the words I wanted to say; she was yelling what I couldn't. It was as if she could feel my anguish and send it out. After a time, I found my voice and was able to release so much instead of being frozen in my memories, hurt, and shame.

The power of a group, of being witnessed and supported, is truly invaluable for healing.

I want to share another story about the strength of group ritual that is not just about grief and pain.

Fast forward to my life at sixty. I was at a retreat on the Dagara tradition, which was being led by my friend Susan Hough. The Dagara tradition comes from a tribe primarily located in Burkina Faso, West Africa. This particular retreat was being held in Southern France, and the ritual was on the elements of their medicine wheel. We spent each of the five days immersed in a different element and a ritual associated with that element. The fourth day was mineral. Mineral is about our stories.

Before I started this retreat, I had been searching for my next step in life. I was separating from my husband and looking for a new direction. I always wanted to write, but because of my dyslexia and not learning to read or spell above a first-grade level until I was seventeen, I figured that wouldn't happen. On this particular day, the ritual was about letting go of old stories and letting the minerals fill us with our new ones.

A few weeks before, I had been introduced to the writing program The Author Incubator by random chance. I applied, and they said if my application was accepted for review I would receive a text for an interview in a week. Well, two weeks went by. I had not heard anything, so I figured that wasn't the direction I was supposed to be going in.

I left for France feeling a little disappointed but looking forward to the week.

Guess what happened? During the mineral ritual, I distinctly got the sense my stories were changing. I felt alive and exuberant. When we got back to the retreat center from our mineral ritual, I decided randomly to dress up for dinner. I even put a little make-up on and did my hair. That was not the norm for me.

About ten minutes after I finished, I received a text asking if I was available for an interview in the next ten minutes with someone from the writing program! It was a FaceTime interview with a full view of me while I was looking good and feeling confident.

Needless to say, this book is the outcome from the interview.

Ritual and ceremony change us and what we are ready for in our lives. They help us release what no longer serves our growth and happiness and fill us up on what does.

I included stories here that don't have anything to do with abuse because healing from abuse also includes finding our path in life. It pushes us to rewrite our stories to ones that are positive and support us and fill our hearts with hope and joy again. Rituals and ceremonies do all of that and more. They help us learn to trust ourselves and others; they help us build confidence and take responsibility for our own lives.

Chapter 3

Why This Process

From the previous chapter, you can see how ritual and ceremony can really help people to move forward quicker and heal at such deep levels. I have studied many traditions over the last forty years. One of them, the Dagara medicine wheel which I learned through Sobonfu Somé, has been one that resonated deeply with me. I believe this is because of the people that make up the Dagara. They are kind and open. Even though their lives include a lot of struggle, they are always present and clear with their communications. But I think most of all there are two beliefs that I hold dear and learned from them the most.

First, everyone (and I mean everyone) is considered a gift to the community. Everyone is born into the world to bring their special gift. They are honored and welcomed from conception. If someone is born with an abnormality as we in the West would call it, the village doesn't scorn them, put them in special classes, or on drugs. The village recognizes as a community this person was brought in to teach them, that there is something the village must learn. So they embrace them and love them and work to understand what they and the village need.

Secondly, even if you have no genetic relation to people in the village, you are considered a wife or husband, sister or brother, aunt or uncle, mother or farther, grandmother or grandfather, or the child. They recognize everyone as closely related. Sobonfu used to tell stories of when she needed a certain kind of support for a problem she had or wanted something specific for dinner, she would find the person who could provide it and spend the day or night with them. She specifically remembers that at age five when she found out she only had one biological mother, she didn't believe them. She truly thought she had many mothers. In a five-year-old's mind, that is very conceivable.

In terms of my own challenges with childhood abuse, one thing about the Dagara that stands out so strongly for me is that in their language there is no word for abuse. I remember asking Sobonfu why. Her answer was simple and profound:

They simply do not have any abuse in the villages. Every person is responsible for everyone else. When there is a problem in the village, many people help; when you are sad, people love you and listen to you. When children get into mischief, they don't call them out and punish them. They realize that once the child recognizes that maybe they shouldn't have done something, they can always correct it. There is always a way to make things better.

Those are the reasons I was able to heal, primarily using this tradition, at such a deep level. It's an amazing feeling to finally know that I am a gift, and so are you and your clients. We all have something unique that only we can do. And our experiences, no matter what they are, have shaped us into the person needed to bring those gift into the world.

I would recommend taking the time to read Welcoming Spirit Home: Ancient African Teachings to Celebrate Children and Community by Sobonfu Somé.

I also use rituals that I learned in other traditions because of the value they bring to my life. I have studied indigenous traditions for forty years. They all have wonderful healing and transformative value.

When we have been severely abused as children, we cannot recognize that we have a gift, let alone find a purpose to our exitance or even find a vision for life. In the Dagara tradition, our fire element may have been put out or is so ignited that we are full of rage—it is out of balance.

In a Christian tradition, this could relate to losing the vision god has for us, not seeing any longer that we are here because god loves us and has a plan for us.

The scars of abuse can stop use from feeling safe or having balance with our emotions, especially when we start the process of healing. The grief that takes over can be so overwhelming. In the Dagara tradition, I would want to do a water ritual to let go and let my emotions flow instead of stopping them up. Going to the waters to heal and be renewed is spoken of throughout the bible. What if you could create a ritual around this for your Christian clients?

Feeling safe in our own bodies is non-existent for many who have been abused. We can get lost by identifying as a victim or feeling like a victim so that we lose our true identity. We are not able to feel the nurturing of the earth element in the Dagara tradition. What if you could learn to create a ritual in your client's tradition that helps them feel safe in their bodies and help them learn to love being human again?

Sometimes, the stories we have of ourselves are so distorted that they can make honest communication difficult. Trusting ourselves and others can be hard to come by. Is there a sacred way you can help your clients release or change these stories?

Last but not least, the joy and magic of life can be lost behind the masks we wear. The ability to transform, let go of these masks, and draw from our authentic self can be scary. We are stuck and uncomfortable with change. What would a ritual in your client's tradition look like?

When we balance the elements inside our psyche, our life becomes more balanced. Carl Jung has many books on this. One of my favorite quotes of his is, "Who looks outside dreams, who looks inside awakens." Most traditions have these elements, and they can be incorporated into rituals and ceremonies to meet your client's needs.

For this book, I have organized rituals from multiple traditions into a pattern that I know works. The pattern is:

1. Finding home—This is about being comfortable in our skin, reuniting with our own spirit, our hearts, and our bodies. We start to identify with the kinder side of ourselves instead of the judgmental side. We learn to ground in our hearts and be present, as well as learn to recognize when we have separated from our hearts. It is also about what our identity is.

2. Releasing—This is learning to have our emotions move and not be stuck, releasing the stories that no longer serve us and forgiving ourselves and those that hurt us or didn't keep us safe.

3. Vision—Finding purpose and passion for life. Sometimes as we heal, we simply want to know what to do next, or we need to understand our purpose in life, have something outside of ourselves that we can focus on for a while or long term that reignites us, and helps us move forward through the process of recovery. It is finding what brings joy into our lives.

4. Honoring Ourselves—This one is big. In the process of recovery, many of us have to transform and change so many things with in us, including the way we think, the way we perceive others and ourselves. Go from victim to warrior to wise woman strong in herself. Speak her truth and ask for what she wants. Remove the masks that she hides behind. These rituals are for that purpose.

Your clients may be at different stages of their recovery, so it is completely appropriate to start a client with rituals that meet them where they are. If you have someone who is really stuck in their emotions, you may want to try one of the release rituals. Some people I have known need to have a vision to go to before they can let go of their grief.

A big key to incorporating ritual into your practice is to really understand that using your intuition is so important. You know your clients; you have been working with them closely. You will know what they are comfortable with, when you can push them gently out of their comfort zone, and you will know when to push the boundaries of your own comfort zone.

When learning the processes in this book, it can be very helpful to have one or two others that you are comfortable with, other therapists, friends, or people that want to learn this with you, to support you, and practice these rituals with them before you introduce them to your clients. If you have practiced ritual and ceremony in your own life and are comfortable with it, then jump in and introduce these to your clients.

Introducing Ritual to Your Clients

"Ritual is to the soul what physical food is to our bodies." -Sobonfu Somé

"Your Sacred space is where you can find yourself again and again." -Joseph Campbell

Carl Jung expresses ritual and ceremony as important to mark the transitions of our lives. Without it, people suffer deeply. Ritual and ceremony create a bridge between our past and present, making it easier to honor the good and the bad. It gives us the ability to bridge the conscious and unconscious to create greater healing and awareness of the divine.

Ritual has been used by all cultures and religions forever. They are not owned by any one group, and we create our own to bring comfort and a sense of safety and growth into our lives.

If you are working with clients who have been traumatized by ritual, then call it a process. For those who find comfort in religion, talk about the rituals of their religion and how these new rituals complement those.

One of my dear friends was in a real mess in her twenties. She was experiencing abusive relationships, doing lots of partying, and had young children whom she would leave alone at night when she went out. Sometimes, she would bring strangers home that she met while out at night. It was just a mess.

I prayed that she would find something to help her. She did. She became born again in Christ, and it changed her life for the better.

However, it also changed our relationship. She could no longer accept my beliefs and what I was teaching about spirituality and ritual, which was not Christianity. We ended up not speaking for many years.

Once when I knew I would be in the town she lived, I called, and we decided to catch up. One of the interesting things I found out was she and a few other women met regularly to do rituals in Christ's name. One was a fire ritual that I had taught before but had never paired a particular religious doctrine with it. They would write the names of those they needed to forgive, their name being the first, and prayed for Jesus to help them. Then they burned the letters in a sacred fire built while they prayed.

This is a great example of how to introduce a non-doctrine-specific ritual into a specific doctrine. My friends group basically took a ritual where fire is the catalyst for releasing and put it into their Christian beliefs. If you have a client that believes they are atheist, this is a simple forgiveness ritual; if Hindu, this could be to Vishnu, the most compassionate one. If your client follows nature traditions, such as Wiccan, this is a fire ritual.

All the rituals in this book can be translated into most doctrines and belief systems. This is where you trust your intuition and judgement so you can really aid your clients recovery using rituals and ceremonies. You know your clients!

Start with easy and simple rituals. Write the meditations in your own words, and start guiding your clients through them. Get a small group together, and do the water releasing ritual. It is simple, yet extremely powerful. The rituals in this book are supportive and healing, powerful yet really gentle. Rituals create a sacred and safe environment when done well.

Chapter 4

How Does Ritual Work?

B efore we can get into the steps of my process, it's important for you to understand how ritual works; without this basic understanding, you will never be able to use ceremonies and rituals effectively.

It has been known for a really long time that the mind can be your ally or it can stop us in our tracks from changing. For the purposes of this book, I am referring to the mind as the conscious mind or the thinking mind. This is the one that we use to make conscious decisions, to have conversations with ourselves, and to make decisions on what to do next. The subconscious mind is the place where the beliefs that we live by but are not aware of reside.

For example, someone who stays in an abusive relationship consciously knows they should leave, but they don't. This is an example of the subconscious belief that it is safer with the danger they know than the danger of changing to something they don't know. Their friends may be saying, "*Why* do you stay?" But if their friends weren't raised to believe they deserve to be abused, then their subconscious doesn't hold the belief, and they have a hard time understanding their friend's behavior.

There has been so much research in the last few decades on the mind, conscious and subconscious, and the brain. I find it interesting that science still can't find the physical place where the mind and consciousness reside in the physical brain. I remember when I was in high school studying biology, the scientific theories back then said that the brain was limited in the way it grew, that it stopped changing when we became adults, and continued to lose cells as we aged. Communication of brain cells was mostly fixed and linear, hard-wired. Basically, it was limited, and we couldn't change our behaviors once we became adults.

Wow, has that scientific theory changed with time! Now we understand how little we really know. The brain is very plastic and adaptable. One neuron can communicate over many pathways to multiple other neurons, and those pathways are three-dimensional in their communication. They can create new neural pathways when some get damaged. Behaviors and abilities like speech and motor skills that have been lost because of damage can be learned to be done by a different part of the brain.

We also know that the reality of the mind, especially the subconscious, can be changed without necessarily bringing the dark thoughts to the surface and analyzing them and reliving the traumas. I recently read that we can discuss a trauma three times and be fine, but on the fourth, we start to retraumatize ourselves, that the subconscious really can't distinguish between old events and what is happening now in the moment. The subconscious interprets them as all in the present, the now. This is especially true in young children. If you will recall during the events of 9/11, when the media was constantly replaying the destruction of the Twin Towers, there was a call by the American Association of Pediatrics to stop airing the footage. The difference between the children and the adults is that adults' rational minds could say, "This is a repeat." Children's minds can't. Additionally, we know that even as adults, our subconscious was still traumatized.

The Dalai Lama has worked closely with scientists to open up the study of the brain and the mind with monks that had been meditating for decades. Wolf Singer, the director of the Max Planck Institute for Brain Research in Frankfurt, Germany said, "Meditation is a highly active mental state." He described studies indicating that certain brain waves become synchronized when a person's mind is attentive—or meditating—that areas of the brain thought to be active only while sleeping are active during conscious meditation.

Science has learned that traits and behaviors previously thought to be hard to change are affected by ritual and ceremony and can be changed more quickly. Those suffering with P.T.S.D. and other psychological challenges can use these tools to heal. Science has shown that we can calm the sympathetic nervous system through these practices and find solutions that teach our minds to take us into those states easily.

Treatments such as A.I.T. and E.F.T. have been developed so we can actually reprogram the conscious and subconscious mind.

The interesting thing about all this science is that indigenous peoples and their healers and shamans have intuitively known for centuries that the mind isn't healed through talking and reliving the traumas but that it is healed when we let go of them, that ritual, ceremony, and deep meditation—the processes that take us deep inside and connect us with our own psyche—are what heal us and that we connect to higher realms of consciousness in these processes. Through ritual and ceremony, we bypass the analytical mind and go to the deeper parts of our being.

Why Community

There is an old saying that it takes a village to raise a child. It also takes a village to heal from abuse and trauma. However, if our personal community—family, family friends, or our church—were involved with the abuse and covering it up, we don't feel safe at all there. That is why it is important to find those that support us.

For me, it was through friends and my therapist that I found communities and groups to support my healing. These were, and still are, women's groups that come together to back each other both for support and ritual. Some were groups I met through the people like Sobonfu Somé that I studied their traditions with. The power of a group is that they hear you, witness you, and support you while healing. It also gives so much to the group to witness someone else's transformation and healing. For many who have suffered from abuse, seeing others heal can help them to have confidence that they can heal and see that there is hope for the future.

Also, the energy of people coming together to witness one another is powerful. Each person lends their uniqueness. They can feel how they contribute and gain inner strength from helping one another. Miraculous things can happen.

Additionally, it takes the burden off of you as the therapist to be the soul leader in someone's healing. When groups come together in ritual and ceremony, everyone supports everyone else. It starts by creating the space for the ritual and includes helping each other through the process. By all being involved at different levels, each person learns more about being responsible for their own healing and serving others. People love to help one another. I believe our true nature is kindness and generosity toward one another, but because of the abuse we suffered from those that loved us and cared for us, we have learned to mistrust. In ritual and ceremony, we can learn to trust one another again.

I have been in many rituals where there are people of all kinds of faith and races. I remember one specifically where great healing happened with three people who were on the opposite side during World War II. One of the families were soldiers of the Nazi party and the other was from concentration camps. These people had all the right to mistrust, yet they learned to trust and heal.

I personally healed deeply during a ritual where my sister was with me. We had always had a rough relationship, and she was one of my close family that allowed the abuse to happen to avoid being abused herself; we were very young, and her behavior is truly understandable. During this ritual and because of the support from others present, we were able to go very deep inside and heal the wounds. I was able to completely forgive her and she me. This could have taken years in traditional counseling. However, it took only a few hours in ritual.

Overview of the Process

For most of us when we go to a ceremony such as a wedding or even a funeral, we know what to expect. There will be a place such as a church. There will be flowers, places to sit, and someone to lead the ceremony. Within the ceremony, there will be familiar rituals like reading from the Bible or other sacred books. Prayer, reflection and meditation, communion. And there will be a close to the ceremony that is recognizable that this ceremony is over.

This chapter is the "how to" guide and is written for those of you reading this book that have never facilitated rituals and ceremonies. If you have done them before, look at this chapter as a reminder. There is a checklist in the appendix. After years of doing this work, I still like my checklist.

Ritual is about flow within structure. This chapter gives you the overall structure of ritual. The following chapters give you the understanding of the different types I recommend and their unique contribution so you can learn to flow within the structure. As you learn each ritual, you will gain understanding and confidence, and your rituals will start to flow easily.

You can start with a group meeting in your office one evening a week. Pick a different meditation every week and guide your clients through it, and then have them share what they experienced. You can use the structure laid out in the rest of this chapter. This will give your clients a feel for the process before you have them join you for a longer ritual.

Pre-Ritual

Once the date is set for the ritual, you are actually being worked by the ritual about a week beforehand. In other words, your subconscious gets excited and starts working, processing what will happen.

Have you ever noticed a few days before a wedding, the couple can get really nervous that little things may not go so smoothly, have second thoughts, or forget to pack something important? In the west, we attribute this to nerves. Indigenous people attribute it to the internal soul changes that are starting. It's the beginning of letting go so we can be altered internally and take our next step forward. This really is a good thing, but it can be uncomfortable. All you have to do is simply take notice.

There is a ritual known as grief ritual in the Dagara tradition. It is one of my favorites and most powerful for transforming. However, because it is so strong, I've noticed that I have to be very self-aware for about a week before because I can get grumpy, forgetful, and start finding reasons not to go. Once there, especially when we are setting up the space, my need for control comes out. People who I love will start to irritate me. I start to think, "Why am I even doing this?" and I get frustrated. Then inevitably my friend Susan will come over and say, "Yup, ritual has started!" I will agree, laugh, and pull myself together again.

The steps for facilitating ritual and ceremony:

1. Creating the space
2. Opening invocation
3. Performing the ritual and or ceremony
4. Closing the space
5. Returning home after the ritual

Creating sacred space

You know how there are places you walk into and they just feel good? They feel safe and welcoming. This is what you will want to create!

1. The Setting

The first step is finding a place that has this feeling and is big enough for those you will be working with.

For one-on-one or a small group, your office may work. If the weather is good, a private place outside can be really lovely, especially for releasing rituals. Space at retreat centers, hotels, and even private houses are nice. Many churches are very welcoming to this kind of work. Turning a ritual that is only a few hours into an overnight retreat can be very successful by giving the participants the time to integrate the ritual before reentering their daily lives.

If you are renting a space, you will want to make sure that burning candles, incense, and sage are okay with the management and that there is not a restriction on noise. For example, some retreat centers have rules for silence at night. If you are staying overnight and the place provides the meals, know the times and rules. We used to go to a lovely retreat center; however, they were very strict about meal times, and that caused us a challenge more than a few times once we were in the flow of the ritual!

If there are other guests at the facility, make sure that your area is private.

2. *Clearing the Energy*

The second step can be done before your clients get there or with them. For shorter rituals, I suggest you have most of the setup done. For longer ones, it is nice to have the participants help with the setup. It gives them a sense of belonging, community, and safety.

First, you will want to clear the energy in the room. I suggest doing this before your clients arrive. It is a time that can help you get centered and grounded. This can be done by using sage or sacred incense such as nag champa. Light whatever you are using and walk around the room, visualizing anything negative leaving the room and the room being filled with love.

When I am in a place that doesn't allow the use of fire, I may use a light essential oil such as lemon or orange. Lavender is nice, too, and you can get sage and palo santo essential oils. I'd avoid anything strong; just a drop in each corner of the room with the intention to clear the room and bring in peace and love works great.

3. Deciding the Setup

Next, decide the setup. The setups for each ritual are described in the chapters pertaining to that type of ritual. This is the overview of the processes.

There will be at least one focal point, such as an altar, an area to sit, stand, or lay down, and possibly an area where people will be making something. Once you have decided where everything goes, it is time to set up.

If the participants are helping with the setup, once everyone has arrived and settled, have each person go around the circle and say their name and have the group say back "Welcome, (their name)." You can then have them briefly share why they are there.

Next, explain to them what you will be doing and what you want them to do. It is important to be patient and clear. Remember, they are already in the process and will forget some of what you tell them and get it mixed up. This is why I love checklists. Over time, if you work with mostly the same people, a core group will start to form that becomes familiar and comfortable with the steps and will naturally help you and know what to do, even if you forget.

Creating the Focal Point

Focal points, sometimes referred to as altars and shrines, are where we come to alter our self and honor life. We build shrines publicly to honor others all the time. We can build personal ones to honor those we love and ourselves on our journey from abuse to wholeness. We build them in ceremony and ritual to honor the process and elements that will be helping us, just like how the altar in a Christian church honors Christ.

These can be as simple or elaborate as you want. When building in a group for longer ritual and ceremony, let the participants build the altars organically. That way they can really feel they are part of the ritual. When they are built spontaneously, they will each have a unique beauty that is perfect.

Some basic guidelines are:

Have whoever is building the altar say an opening prayer asking for guidance from their higher self, god, angels, the elements, their guides, etc. It should be whatever feels right for the belief systems of the participants. For example, when I am with my Peruvian teachers, we call in the four directions, mother earth, and father sky. In a Christian ritual, it could be Jesus; if Catholic, then maybe mother Mary and the angels.

Use flowers, unscented candles and cloths that relate to the ceremony. For example, if it is a releasing ceremony, use water and the color of blue. The shrine can be on a table, the floor, or both for dimension.

If you have had the participants bring objects with them, they can place those on the altar at this time if appropriate. More details for each ritual and ceremony are in the chapters that follow.

The final step is placing the chairs, pillows, and comfortable places to lay down where you want them as relates to the ritual.

If you did the setup prior to the participants arriving, once they arrive and have settled, have each person go around the circle and say their name and have the group say back "Welcome (their name)." You can then have them briefly share why they are there. Once this is done, you will want to explain the purpose of the ritual and the basic flow.

Opening Invocation

The invocation is to help everyone become present and grounded. The invocation is where as a group we call on guidance from god, the angels, the elements, ancestors, whatever belief system you are using or a combination when people of different beliefs are present.

If you have some in the group who have done this with you, have them participate. Before the invocation, have them choose or you can assign what they will invoke. For example, someone of the Christian belief may call in the holy trinity, nature beliefs—the animals and elements.

Have everyone stand if they can during this processes.

You will want to use wording specific to the ritual. For example, if it is a ritual for releasing, ask help to know what we want to release most, which is what is no longer needed and is holding us back. This is a time to trust your intuition. I have said things during an invocation or others have said something and my mind went, "Really? Why would you say that?" And later had someone tell me I had said the perfect thing, or I realized I needed to hear what someone else had said.

The Ritual

It is important that you spend time contemplating the ritual to get a true understanding of its purpose before facilitating it.

This way you will be comfortable with the process. The processes are detailed in the following chapters.

Many of the rituals may have a guided meditation. You may want to write these in your own words so they are more familiar to you. Add the time you want to pause in between the questions in the guided meditations. I sometimes write "Take three breaths" or "Count to thirty" in parentheses to remind myself to pause. Time is very different for the person guiding compared to the persons being guided.

In writing, the guided meditations where I wait a few moments means to give them time to do what you have just suggested to them.

If the room is bright and they are comfortable with being blindfolded, they can use a scarf or cloth to cover their eyes.

These meditations are written as if your clients are women. That is simply for ease and consistency. If you are working with men or in mixed sex groups make sure to change the pronouns to support them.

Also understand that the flow may change some in different situations. You may want to add or take a step out. Once you have done ritual a couple of times, you will have a greater understanding of this and find what works best for you as the facilitator. The very nature of using ritual and ceremony to heal will make the experience more fluid as you learn to meet the needs of the group and yourself.

It is also important for you to participate in the ritual. This is very comforting to the participants.

Closing the Ritual

Once you have gone through the ritual, it is important to close the space. This is done through an invocation following the same pattern as the opening, but this time you are thanking those whose help you have invoked. Ask for continued guidance over the next few weeks as we integrate all that has happened.

If you have done a releasing ritual, for example one of the ones using water, you will want to take the water and pour it out on the earth and leave the bowls in the sun for few days or sprinkle them with salt so the energy can be cleared. Any rituals requiring something additional being done with the items will be mentioned as part of the details of the ritual.

Returning Home After the Ritual

Ritual is very powerful for bringing change into our lives. Just because the physical ritual is done doesn't mean we aren't still processing especially on a subconscious level. The participants, including you, will want to take care of themselves for a few days after.

Drink a lot of water to clean the system and remind us to keep flowing with the process. Take salt baths, eat nourishing food, and spend some time integrating. These are all wonderful ways to nurture ourselves. Writing every day in a journal to acknowledge the changes and insight is very helpful.

You and your clients are in an altered state for a day or so depending on the length and depth of the ritual. Because of being in an altered state, pay attention to your dreams. Walks in nature, swimming in the ocean, doing fun and gentle activities that feel good are great.

Pay attention to nature and the messages and symbols that it is showing you.

It is best to avoid recreational drugs or alcohol for at least twenty-four hours and preferably no violent or disturbing TV/movies. Because of the altered state, the effects can be heightened. Parties and large crowds right after ritual can also be more intense.

Ritual puts us in a receptive mode, so the more we spend time in positive and nurturing environments, the more we will receive from the ritual.

You may want to schedule a group meeting a week or two after the ritual to have people check in with each other. It is amazing how many similarities they will find in their experiences.

Preparing Yourself for Facilitating

Here are some of the tasks you can do to prepare to facilitate ritual.

1. Write the meditations in your own words and according to the group's needs.

2. Spend time contemplating the purpose of the ritual and the steps you will be following. I always have notes handy. Remember you will also be in an altered state.

3. Learn a grounding technique if you don't already have a way to center yourself. An easy one is to visualize your feet are roots sinking into the ground below you and the earth is holding you and giving you energy. Practice it so you can ground yourself in any circumstance. There is a meditation in the next chapter, finding home, where you find your grounding cord.

4. Because of your background as a therapist or counselor, you are used to "holding space" for others as they process. In ritual, you will be doing the same thing but on a bigger scale. The energy during ritual can be stronger, so really grounding and staying focused is essential.

5. If the energy of the ritual feels low, you may have to bring it up. If it feels unfocused, you may be the one to bring it back into focus. Learn to track the energy and keep it balanced.

6. If you have someone that you are comfortable with, it will be nice to have their support. That way they can help track where everyone is in the process especially for the longer rituals.

7. Make sure you eat well, drink water to stay hydrated, and get plenty of rest for a few days and especially the night before.

8. You may be surprised how after the ritual you are hungry or you may feel tired. For longer rituals, have food already prepared for you or do take out. Take the next day off when you are first learning to do the longer rituals. Follow the same advice you will give the participants.

9. Some rituals will feel great and be energizing to you. Still follow the guidelines laid out in Returning Home After the Ritual above.

If you have never been involved in ritual, go to some yourself. Create a group of friends and peers to learn with. Do the personal rituals and see how they feel before recommending to your clients. Most of all, learn to trust yourself and have fun.

To Recap:

Ritual and ceremony have been used through the ages to help heal, and research now agrees that it works. There are five basic steps to most rituals: clearing the energy of the place, building a focal point or altar, invoking help from what we perceive guides us and helps us, the actual ritual, and then closing the space. Additionally, it is important for you as the facilitator to prepare for the ritual and for you and the participants to care for yourselves afterward.

Knowing the structure allows for you to flow freely and confidently through the ritual.

Chapter 5

Finding Home

F inding home is about being comfortable in your "skin," reuniting with the spirit, the heart, and the body. Starting to identify with the kinder side of yourself instead of the judgmental side. Finding home is learning to ground in your heart and be present, as well as learning to recognize when you have separated from your heart, your nurturing side.

It is also about feeling safe with yourself. Many who have been abused have learned to trust others before they trust themselves. This can be disastrous because much of the time we are still around abusive people who don't have our best interest at heart. The opposite can also be true. They might say, "I will trust no one but myself," yet they don't have a kind relationship with themselves. They continue to abuse the child within.

Finding home is also learning to nurture yourself. It's about physically liking the body you have and the way you look: nurturing your body, resting when needed, exercising at the right times, eating the right foods, learning to listen to the body and what it needs, letting yourself play.

It helps you to be emotionally aware of yourself; when you're anxious or scared, do you listen to yourself or blow it off? Do you acknowledge when you're sad or grieving, or are you simply confused about what you are feeling? Can you be okay with your emotions? Do you understand the link between your physical body and emotions? Can you self-regulate when in a stressful situation?

Emotionally, do you feel strong and empowered when interacting with others or making decisions about what is best for you? Can you say yes when it is right and no when it is not?

This last part is especially important for those who have been abused. Many times we are too afraid to speak what is in our hearts. We are uncomfortable in our body or may even feel the body betrayed us. By becoming grounded and trusting ourselves as our own authority, we can start to find comfort again.

Rituals and Meditation

Meditation

Finding your heart and creating a safe place for you and your inner child

This meditation is to help your clients feel their whole body and become present with it, to learn to regulate their breathing using a count of three in and five out, and to find a safe place inside themselves. It is best to do sitting.

Meditation Dialogue: Items in parentheses are for you to do, not part of what you will say while facilitating this meditation. Small and long pauses are relative to the time you have for the meditation and your clients ability to stay present with you. Too fast and they don't have time to process and do what you just said. Too long and they will be distracted.

Meditation Dialogue

"Get comfortable siting. Take a breath in and out (small pause).

Feel the surface holding you. Whether that is a chair, the floor, a couch. Feel it supporting you (small pause).

Let yourself sink in and feel really comfortable. Feel gravity supporting you and giving you a sense of being held in gentle arms (small pause).

Take another deep breath in and out (small pause).

I want you to put your left hand on your breast bone with your palm in the center. Feel your chest expanding as you breathe in and coming back in when you breathe out (small pause).

Keeping your left hand where it is, take your right hand and place it just below your navel. See if you can sense the movement of your breath in and out with both hands (small pause).

Can you feel the warmth of your body through your clothes (small pause)?

Now I want you to start to breathe in to the count of three and out to the count of five (do a couple of breaths, counting slowly for them pacing their breathing, then give them a moment to do a few on their own).

Now I want you to see if you can feel the edges of your body where your skin meets your clothes (small pause)?

Can you feel the air coming in your nose and your lungs expanding, your belly moving? In for three; out for five (small pause).

Now feel the edges of your body again where your clothes touch your skin (small pause).

Now feel where your body connects with gravity. Feel your feet on the ground (small pause), the backs of your legs connecting the with the surface you are sitting on (small pause).

Your sit-bones and spine supporting your neck and head and arms (small pause).

Now imagine a cord as wide as you want extending down from your heart area just under your left hand, extending down your spine through your pelvis, through your thighs and calves, out the bottom of your feet into the earth. It can be as wide as you want. Maybe it extends from your pelvis directly to the earth incorporating your legs and feet (small pause).

Feel this cord go as deep as you like maybe even to the center of the earth, extending through all the layers. Feel it branch out like the roots of a tree if you like, anchoring you firmly in the earth (small pause).

Like the roots of a tree this is your grounding cord. It is always available to you; you simple have to think of it and feel it tap into the earth. This cord is here to help you feel centered, safe, and nurtured. You can call on it anytime you want (small pause).

Now feel the nurturing energy of the earth come up the cord, filling your feet and legs and pelvis with gentle energy. Maybe it has a color or temperature, maybe you feel it tingle or vibrate (small pause).

Feel this energy connect with the hand on your belly as it moves up to your heart area just under your left hand (small pause).

Feel this whole area fill with this grounding and nurturing energy that is uniquely yours. Feel it fill your whole body bringing you home to you (small pause).

Your body is your home here on earth. It wants to take care of you (small pause).

It is always here with you, trying its best to do whatever you ask, taking the best care of you it can. Your body is always with you. It can be your best friend (small pause).

Now take a deep breath in and out, feeling your lungs fill with air. How does that feel (small pause)?

Our body is the best tool we have to knowing what is going on with our emotions in any given moment. When you are relaxed and breathing easy, like right now, how do you feel (small pause)?

Really notice how your arms and legs and hips feel; notice how soft and relaxed are your belly your shoulders (small pause)?

Now just for a moment, think of having to slam on your brakes while driving your car to avoid something. Can you feel the change in your breath? Faster, shorter. What has happened in your belly (small pause)?

Now feel your grounding cord again, take a slow breath in and even slower out. Count three in and five out (small pause).

Notice how you feel, how you can use your breath to regulate your emotions, bring you back to a safe and nurturing place within yourself (small pause).

Now feel your body, especially your heart and belly under your hands, and ask your body if there is anything it wants you to know to help you feel more connect (longer pause)?

What does your body want to feel: healthier and stronger (longer pause)?

What can you do, starting today, to nurture your relationship with your body (longer pause)?

Now thank your body for whatever it shared with you and know that you will remember this. Even if you feel you didn't hear anything, know that something will come when the time is right. Promise to do the best you can to fulfill these desires (small pause).

Now feel your grounding cord. Know deep in your heart that it is always there, and you can consciously connect to it any time you choose by placing your hand on your heart and belly or simply by thinking of your cord (small pause).

Now take a few deep breaths in, becoming aware of your toes and feet, your legs, hips, belly, and chest. Your arms, your back, your neck and head. Wiggle your fingers and toes (small pause).

When you are ready, gently open your eyes, staying in this quiet and nurturing space, and write in your journal what you learned and what your body desires in this moment.

Post-Meditation

Remind your clients to check in every day upon waking and before they sleep to connect with the cord they just learned and to see what their body wants to be healthy and strong that day.

If you want to turn this into a group ritual, you can have them share at the end of writing. You can make it longer by having them do a drawing in addition to the writing, and at the end, have them share their experience with the group. This meditation is also nice to do with other rituals on a longer day or weekend retreat. Perhaps you can pair this with an earth mandala (explained in the next section). Have them build the earth mandala to represent their body, and then after the mediation, go back to it and add items or remove or rearrange the items in it. Then do the next ritual and check out the mandala again. Remember at the end of the entire retreat to have them thank what they learned from the mandala and gently dismantle it.

Earth Mandala Ritual

The formal definition of the word mandala is a spiritual and ritual symbol representing the universe. An earth mandala, for the purposes of this book, is a physical structure you build on the earth to symbolize where we are personally right now. The items it is built of represent how we feel right now, what we want to change, a question we are asking answers for, or things we want to change in our present situations. They should inspire deeper insights. They can be personal or communal, large or small.

These kinds of circles have been traced to almost all cultures. I first learned about earth mandalas studying with a Peruvian teacher. The key is it is a symbolic representation that our subconscious can gather meaning from.

They are created outside on the earth. They are generally one to one-and-a-half feet in diameter and have a boundary (generally circular in shape), and items are placed inside the of the circle.

I have seen the boundary built of sticks, flowers with their stems on, stones, and even shells found while building them on the beach. The boundary represents the edges of our personal universe. The inside is what we are seeking.

For example, if you are incorporating an earth mandala with a retreat on releasing our old stories and finding our new ones, when the mandalas are first built, they can contain items that represent the stories we want to release, always add something for the stories you don't yet know you want to release. The item can represent the triggers still felt. For example, sticks that the person asks to represent their fear of being around men or the fear they still hear when there is a noise at night they can't identify and takes them back into their memory.

After the releasing ritual, they will want to remove those items and return them to nature away from their mandala as a symbolic gesture of releasing the old story and then put items that are beautiful and joyful to represent the new story they want to create inside the circle before the next ritual of creating their new story.

At the end of the retreat, have them dismantle the mandala by giving all the items back to nature. That is why they are built out of items that come from nature.

I have kept some of the items I have put in earth mandalas I have built that represent the positive changes and answers I have sought.

For personal earth mandalas I have done on my own, I have kept mine open for days, returning to them at least once a day to observe the changes and make changes myself. I have built them in the woods, in fields, and my gardens. Always away from where other humans might disturb them. I found sometimes I have put food or seeds in my earth mandalas, and they disappeared into nature. I even had one where a bird left its droppings! In one of the traditions I study, this is considered a blessing. The bigger the better!

Building an Earth Mandala

Time Needed: Whether this is part of a group of rituals or a personal mandala, the initial setup is half an hour to an hour. If done with multiple rituals, like the one described above, fifteen minutes every time they visit the mandala and fifteen to close it. If this is one they are building on their own, they can spend as much time as they want meditating while sitting near their mandala, writing in their journals, or simply relaxing and asking more questions and then listening for the answers.

Purpose: Understanding the purpose or intent for the mandala is important. Is this one to get an answer to a question? If so, they really need to form the question and ask for specific guidance during the invocation and creating the space, as well as bring that question to mind every time they go to the mandala. Do they have something they want guidance on to change in their life like the habit of over eating when they are stressed? Forming the intention and then building the mandala is critical so they can use it as a focus

Materials Needed: Depending on the purpose or intention of the mandala, they may want to bring with them an item that represents that purpose or intention like a favorite flower, seeds, or candy. If they are bringing something like a picture, they have to remember this will be left outside and unless protected could be damaged. That is why simply finding natural items as representations is easiest.

Steps:

1. Have the participants go outside and find a place they are drawn to that will be away from others who may tamper with it.

2. Say the invocation, asking for help and guidance for the intention of the mandala and to focus them on the intention.

3. If they haven't brought items with them, have them

look in the area for things they are drawn to that can make the border and items they can put inside to represent their intention.

4. Build the mandala. Clear the space of anything they don't want in it. Build the boundary from the items they have and then place the remaining items within the boundary, saying what each represents.

5. When they are done, if it is a personal mandala, they may want to take a few minutes sitting with it and writing in their journal or just pondering the question or intention for any insights. Once done, leave the mandala where it is, knowing they will be coming back either later that day or the next day. That is why I like to build the personal mandala close to my home or where I hike regularly. I also go on vacation to the ocean and will build one for the duration of the vacation.

6. If this is part of a group of rituals, have them come back to the group for the next ritual, leaving the mandala intact.

7. For personal mandalas, they will want to visit regularly over a few days, noticing any changes while they were gone. They should always ask the question, "What might this change represent?" If they have gotten an answer or insight while they were away, they may want to remove

or add items to the mandala. Spend time contemplating on the question or intention and write about it.

8. If done in a group of rituals, have each participant visit their mandala in between each ritual and make changes that represent how they have changed through the rituals.

9. For personal mandalas, when they feel they have received the answers and insights to their intention, it is time to dismantle their mandala by first saying a closing prayer, thanking all the guidance that has come, the earth for holding the space for their growth and learning, and whatever else they want. Then mindfully return all the items back to the earth so there is no trace of the mandala.

10. If they want, they can take items with them if they have a positive representations.

11. For mandalas that have been part of a group of rituals, they will close them down in the same way after the last ritual of the group.

Ritual for Honoring and Accepting "All of Me"

Time Needed: It is nice to have at least two hours for this for small groups. They really need the time to contemplate and journal. If in a large group, three or four hours is needed to leave time for everyone to share. Limit sharing to five minutes and give at least half hour for their personal time.

Purpose: This ritual is one in which we learn to recognize there are many aspects of ourselves. We are learning to honor all sides of our being and make peace with them—some examples are: the warrior, also known as the masculine, the maiden or feminine side, the inner child, angry side, and victim. Being a kind person, a raging person, smart and beautiful, fat, skinny... The list of possibilities is endless and unique to each of us, although we share many of the same feelings about ourselves. This ritual also helps us to understand that we are not alone in our struggle to accept ourselves. I am always discovering my next level of accepting myself.

I find this ritual most healing, especially in a group, because we can see sides of ourselves in others that we can't see ourselves. Everyone participating in this ritual is a representation of ourselves.

This ritual can seem very vulnerable to the participants, including yourself, yet it is very helpful for your clients to see you open like this.

The basic ritual is this: They will take items from the altar one item at a time that either they brought with them or you provide, come back to their space, place it on the cloth, and ask what aspect of themselves they haven't accepted that this item represents. Then they will write about that. Suggest they write about how that aspect has helped them, caused them problems, how they can find comfort in it, or use it in a good way. As you know, so many see anger as bad. It can be great when used appropriately. For me, it can help me to see that the situation that is causing me to get angry needs to change. I can use the energy to change or lash out. It is my choice. The anger is not good or bad; it is how I use it that can help me or cause me pain.

After they finish each item, they then go back and get another and repeat the process. The purpose is to find out why they haven't accepted it and to accept that reason as acceptable. When they have no more aspects to address, they can sit quietly or go and get one more item to think of to represent a deeper aspect.

Have everyone come back together and share (if they would like to) the things that surprised them. I remember doing this, and one of the things I had not accepted was my own beauty. It used to be easy for me to accept the bad things about me—but the good things? I was kind and intelligent... No way could I accept that. This work really helped me to see all of me over time and accept the good and bad labels I put on myself. I ended up feeling more balanced and accepting of all of me.

At the end of the sharing, have everyone take a moment to sit with their bundles, journal anything they learned from the group, close the bundles, and come back together for the closing.

Materials: You will need items like stones, shells, feathers, and beads. Some should be pretty and some not so nice. They should be things that can represent the sides of us we love, those we reject, and those we don't yet accept. You can have the participants think about this for a week before the ritual and bring their own items and extras to share if they like. They need to be small enough to create a bundle they will keep with them.

You will also want to bring cloth that each person can use to wrap the items in to create their bundle to take with them. It's good to have precut the fabric into two-foot squares. If they have a scarf or cloth they like, have them bring it. They will also need a journal. You may have paper and pens available if they need it.

Pre-setup: For the space, you will want a central altar where the items can be placed. To decorate the alter you can use candles and flowers, they can actually use the flowers as an item for their bundle if they'd like. They also need cloth to cover the altar and enough room for each participant to sit comfortably with a precut cloth in front of them to put the items on and their journals. You may want some chairs and tables for those who can't comfortably sit on the floor.

Steps:

1. Set up. If a short ritual, you will want to have the altar with the items on it and the cloths cut and available

before they get there. For a longer ritual, you can have the clients help with the setup.

2. Clear the space. Use sage, essential oils, or whatever you are comfortable with as learned in Chapter 4.

3. Once everyone has arrived, have them say their name and the group say welcome, followed by their name

4. Explain the purpose and steps of the ritual to the clients.

5. Open the space. Light the candles and say the invocation. In addition to calling in God, Goddess, guides, and others depending on your tradition, call in their higher selves, inner child, and wise woman to guide them and show them what aspects to accept at this time, to love and accept themselves, and to move forward in their lives.

6. If you have already done the grounding cord meditation with this group, take a moment and have them feel their cord. If not, simply ask everyone to take a moment to center, take a few breaths to get grounded, and when they are ready, go to the altar, pick an item, come back to their seat, put it on their cloth, and ask themselves what this represents to them. Then they should write or draw in their journals about what aspect it represents. As they feel complete on one item, they can go get more and repeat the process. When time is up for this part of

the ritual, give them a few minutes to get an item from the altar that represents anything that did not come to the surface during this ritual.

7. Share. Have each person take a few minutes to share what they learned. Was there a particular aspect they were surprised about?

8. When everyone is done, have them close their bundles. They can tie the ends together, fold it, whatever works best, and then say the closing prayer. Thank them for looking so deeply inside.

9. After the ritual, ask them to put their bundles by their bed where they will see it before they sleep and when they first wake up, with the intent to remind them to love and accept all of themselves even if they are not ready to.

10. Over time or in follow up sessions with you, they can add to the bundle or remove items.

This chapter is really fundamental to recovery, especially the grounding cord. So much of recovery, especially when just opening up to the memories and hurt, is about "How do I feel safe?" The only place we are really safe is when we can trust and count on ourselves, have love for ourselves, and learn to regulate our bodies and emotions when we are triggered. Each one of these rituals and meditations provides a tool to use. Our grounding cord and breathing to bring us back to the present. Our bundle that represents all aspects of us and the unique strengths we find in each aspect. Even the earth mandala as a focal point.

Chapter 6

Releasing

R eleasing is about having our emotions move and not be stuck, liberating the stories that no longer serve us and forgiving ourselves and those that hurt us or didn't keep us safe

When we learn to release and not hold on to our emotions, our past, our pain, and our stories, we are free to flow through our lives feeling full and alive.

When we are able to experience the full range of emotion from deep grief to abundant joy without holding on or getting stuck in one, we can learn to stop controlling and being afraid to feel.

When we are stuck in our emotions, they can come out sideways—we overreact to the simplest situations. We read far more into what others are doing, and we stay in fear.

When we learn to flow through our emotions, it is just like sitting next to a calm stream or beautiful and powerful waterfall that reflect our inner being back to us. Reconciliation and peace-making can become part of our life.

When we don't release our old stories, they come out to be reenacted, creating the same situations with different characters. Our subconscious is hoping to heal the old wound. We put our stories on others: "I was abused by a man that was tall and blonde." Now all men tall and blonde trigger us.

I know of a man who had been sexually abused by his older brother. When his oldest son was the same age as his brother when the abuse began, he started coming down hard on his son and wouldn't let him be alone with the younger children. He knew it was just a matter of time before his son acted out. Imagine the trauma this created in the whole family.

You must release the old stories that no longer serve so you can let in the new. We can find peace and harmony this way. Our environment starts to reflect back a positive environment instead of unsafe and scary. We can learn to float above the turbulence of life instead of being dragged down by it. The following rituals and mediations can be done out of sequence but are very strong when done in order. They provide a place to release, forgive, and create our new stories.

Rituals and Meditations

A Place to Go to Let Go

Time needed: This is a ritual that is personal and more of a place-holder rather than something done in a specific time frame—a few minutes once a day for the most part.

Purpose: The purpose of this ritual is to create a focal point outside of your client for the negative emotions they are feeling to go.

Materials: a small bowl, generally blue to represent water, some salt, and water; a place in their home to keep the bowl where it will not be disturbed and is easily accessible.

Ritual: Simply place the bowl of water with some salt in it somewhere in your home, preferably not your bedroom. Set the intention for your grief, sadness, anger, and other emotions that you release through the day to go to this focal point.

Before going to sleep each night, empty the bowl outside on the earth with the intent of the earth transforming the emotions the water has held. Rinse it, fill it with water and some salt, and set it back on the altar, setting the intent again.

If your client is having a particularly intense moment, they can even sit by the bowl and journal their feelings with the intent of the water helping them to flow and not get stuck. At the end of this, they can take the water outside instead of waiting and refill with water and salt. Why keep the grief inside?

Your client can burn the pages in their journal that hold the negative emotions with the intent they be carried to God, Jesus, or whomever they turn to for comfort and be released and healed.

Group Rituals

Releasing and Filling

Time Needed: Depending on the size of the group, about two hours. At a minimum you want about three to five minutes per person for the first part and three to give for each in the second part with ten to fifteen minutes for the middle for the transition to the second part. For example, if you have eight participants, forty plus fifteen plus forty, or at least one hour and thirty-five minutes

Purpose: This ritual is about consciously releasing negative emotions and stories. It can be very powerful as a group to come together and witness what each person wants to release. Many times others will have something that others in the group want to release and hadn't thought of. Additionally, the process for filling after releasing with something they want to bring in is helpful to be witnessed by other.

As the facilitator, you will want to monitor what they say. For example, if someone were to say, "I want to release my life," you will want to coach them to be more specific about what *in* their life they want to release. They probably don't want to release their life itself. The more specific and concrete their words the better. Most of the time, you won't have to say anything.

During the part where we are calling in what we want, if someone is calling in the negative, you may want to gently coach them on their wording and put it in a positive.

There is no right or wrong way to do this.

Materials:

- A small glass for each participant
- A couple of pitchers to hold water
- Salt
- Basket with at least one stone, shell, glass bead, or another small object for each person
    - You can have them bring one of their own. This basket of items can be used for many rituals like the one in the preceding chapter. I know a therapist that has a basket that must have 100 small items in it that she brings to all her workshops so they can absorb the good energy and pass it on to others.
- A small table to place the glasses on and later the basket
- Cloth to cover the table

- At least one candle on the table (blue and white are nice for this ritual)
- Box to put the glasses at the end in for you to clean later

The Space: Because the first part of this ritual is a releasing ritual and you will be using water as the focal point for the release, have easy access to water to fill the pitchers and to the outside where the participants can carry the glasses of water to be emptied on the earth when the first part of the ritual is done.

Steps:

1. Clear the space. Use sage, essential oils, or whatever you are comfortable with as learned in chapter 4.

2. Set up. Cover the table with the cloths and place the candles, glasses, and salt on the table. Place the pitchers of water and basket of stones and items nearby but not under the table. You can stand for the ritual or have seats around the table. If you do not have a table, the floor is fine for the set up as long as everyone can kneel comfortably.

3. Once everyone is settled, have them each say their name and the group welcome them. Then, take a moment to explain the purpose for the ritual and the procedure.

4. Have everyone gather around the table and do the invocation. This invocation is for the releasing of stories, emotions and beliefs that no longer serve, that are

holding us back. Ask for help and guidance from your "higher power," guides, the earth and water for this.

Ritual:

1. One at a time, have each participant come to the table and put about a teaspoon of salt in a glass. Then have them take the pitcher of water, and as they speak what they want to release, have them start to fill the glass. Once they have spoken all that they want to release, have them take the glass back to where they were standing or sitting, and the next person goes. If you have a song for releasing that you like or a sacred song that is easy to sing, you can have those holding the space for the person releasing sing it. When everyone is done, it is nice to add a line about releasing what I don't know yet needs to be released.

2. Once everyone has gone as a group, go outside and have them give the water to the earth thanking the earth and spirit for taking the water and what they released. Have them leave the glass in the box you provided. If possible, leave this outside. If not, bring it in but place away from the table.

3. Next, have each person pick an item from the box and stand in a circle. Going clockwise around the circle, have each person declare what they want to bring in. It can

be peace, joy, understanding, etc., and a new story about themselves like "I am free to heal easily and gently" or "I see myself as whole and healthy," adding something like "Anything that I don't yet know I need for my healing."

4. Once everyone is done, it can be a nice statement to say, "So be it; it is done," and have everyone repeat the statement

5. Have your closing invocation. This prayer is to thank all the help that was with you and that they continue to help everyone realize the new stories of their lives.

Post-ritual: Have your clients pay attention to their emotions and stories that come up over the next week or so. They will be continuing to release and may have new things that present themselves. This is where it is nice if they have the bowl of water in their home as a focal point for these emotions to go to. This ritual is the one discussed at the beginning of this chapter.

Clean up: Wash the glasses in salt water. If you can let them soak overnight, that is even better. Salt is great for clearing negative energy.

Forgiveness Ritual

Time: One to two hours, depending on the group size.

Purpose: Forgiveness can be so freeing but at the same time very heard. Forgiveness is about us letting go even though we may not feel like it. We may want to hold on to the anger toward someone else, and the negative feelings can keep us in a place of being the victim and use up a lot of our energy we could be using for ourselves. God, Jesus, spirit can also be part of this list. I know I was very angry at even the thought of a God who let bad things happen to me when I was so young.

The ritual is simple; basically, each participant will have a list of those they want to forgive, including themselves. They can create this list during the ritual if you have time or before and bring with them. You can also give them about ten minutes to create or you can have them create it as part of the ritual. They will then burn it with prayers for forgiveness.

Materials:

- A place to build a fire (this can be outside or a fireplace)
- Wood, paper, and a lighter (whatever you use to build fires)
- If there is no place for a fire, have a red candle and a metal bucket or container on a heat-proof surface that they can put the paper they are burning into after they light it with the candle
- Fire extinguisher (just in case!)
- Pens and paper

Steps:

1. Clear the space. Using sage or essential oils, clear the energy.

2. Set up. Have the fire ready to light or candle and bucket. Have paper and pens handy.

3. Take a moment for each person to say their name and be welcomed by the group. Then, explain the purpose for the ritual and the procedure.

4. Take some quiet time for everyone to write their list if they didn't do it beforehand. Have everyone take a moment to reflect on the list they brought and add any additional names. I sometimes suggest they have a line for those they forgot to add or don't know they need to forgive. As well as including themselves.

5. Invocation. This ritual is for forgiveness, so the invocation is for help to forgive ourselves and those we see as having wronged us.

6. Light the fire with the intention that the fire will carry your forgiveness to those on the list and each person can be free of the burden that non-forgiveness created in our hearts.

7. One at a time, have them come to the fire or candle, read the list starting by saying "I forgive…," for each person on the list and put it in the fire.

8. Once everyone has gone, have each person say a word or two that they feel forgiveness will give them, especially forgiving themselves. As they speak this, have the group say it back to them.

9. Conduct the closing prayers of thanks.

10. If you have a fire, stay with it until it has gone out. If you used a candle and have the ashes in a metal container, it is nice to empty this on the earth.

Post-ritual: Have the participants notice over the next few days what comes up around forgiveness and write their insights in their journals.

Releasing Meditation (You can change the wording for a specific release such as releasing anger)

Items in ( ) are for you to do, not part of what you will say while facilitating this meditation. Small and long pauses are relative to the time you have for the meditation and your client's ability to stay present with you. Too fast and they don't have time to process and do what you just said. Too long and they will be distracted.

Meditation Dialogue:

Find a comfortable position to either sit or lie down. Make sure you feel supported by the surface you are on whether that is a chair, couch, floor or bed. You may want a blanket to keep warm (small pause).

Take a few deep breaths in and release them with a sigh. As you inhale, feel like you are filling with a soft blue light. As you exhale, feel the cares of the day go away—in with the blue light and out with anything you want to release in the moment (small pause).

A few more breaths in with blue, out with the cares of the day. This is the only place your mind needs to be right now (small pause).

Now feel yourself sitting next to a body of water, sitting close enough that you can touch it. You may be on a bank next to a stream or river, by a waterfall, or on the beach with the ocean gently lapping at your feet (small pause).

Know you are safe and the water is here to listen to you and already knows you as whole and free.

Ask the water to tell you what in this moment can I easily and gently release? What will help me most in this moment to feel closer to the me that is whole and free? (small pause).

Once you hear or feel the answer, thank the water (small pause).

Now I want you to touch the water; you can use your hand or foot, or you can put your whole body in the water—whatever feels comfortable and safe (small pause).

Is the water warm or cool (small pause)?

Flowing softly around you or still (small pause)?

Feel the water fully supporting your hand or foot or body (small pause).

Now feel whatever it is you are ready to release flow from

you into the water, leaving your body and moving into the water (small pause).

Feel whatever it is leaving your body, and thank it for having been with you, for holding the emotions for you and for its willingness to be released into the water and be transformed. You may see little fish come and eat it or a dolphin or sea turtle carry it away, knowing deeply that the water has taken it gladly and is transforming it into clear and positive energy (small pause).

Once you feel you are complete in your releasing, ask the water to fill you with what you need right now, with the new feelings of joy and peace, with the knowing that you are safe, whole and free (small pause).

Ask the water to give you a word, color, or symbol to anchor the new belief (small pause).

Once you have that, take it into your hands and bring your hands to your heart and feel the word, symbol, color, whatever it is enter your heart and fill you. Take it in deeply and feel the healing spread from your heart to every part of your body (small pause).

When you feel complete, thank the water for helping you today and sending you love. Know that you can always return here to the water (small pause).

Start to feel your breath again as it brings in life-giving air (small pause).

Take a few gentle breaths and start to feel your body safe and supported where you are (small pause). Start to hear the sounds around you and feel your body (small pause).

Slowly, when you are ready, open your eyes, get your journal, and write your experience with the water.

Releasing Stories Meditation

Stories are the interpretation of events that have happened in our lives. When we are abused, the stories we create will tend to always have that taint to them, that filter that is from our pain.

It can be a real challenge to not view life's events through those stories. "I'm a victim" can turn into feeling like you are victimized all the time. "I am undeserving" serves to keep us in the old patters because to find someone that treats us nicely is an unfamiliar store.

You know your client's stories sometimes better than they do and can see how they limit and keep them in their comfort zone. We also know that to cling to the comfort zone can make it difficult to heal.

This ritual is great if you can be outside. Maybe make it part of a retreat program.

Find a quiet place to sit. If you can be outside in a place where there are lots of stones, even better. I like to find a large rock to sit on or go into the mountains and be with the old stone outcroppings. If you are inside you can have some stones around you; hold some if you want, and visualize being surrounded by beautiful stones. If you are outside, feel the rocks and minerals your body is touching, and connect with them.

This can be a very powerful meditation for bringing up the stories. If you have someone that is experiencing deep P.T.S.D., you may want to do this one on one with them before they join a group.

Meditation Dialogue:

Take a few deep breaths. Fill your whole body with the life-giving air you are breathing in. When you breathe out, feel your mind quiet. Let go of any thoughts, worries, and responsibilities of the day (small pause).

This is your time to be present with yourself. In and out with your breath (small pause).

Now feel your breathing filling your bones. Feel it filling your spine and your hips. Breathing out any discomfort (small pause).

Now feel your breath filling your leg bones, your long and strong femurs that gives shape to your thigh, the tibia and fibula of your lower legs (small pause).

Feel your breath fill all the little bones that make up your ankles and feet. There are forty bones that make up each foot and ankle. Fill each one (small pause).

Now fill your ribs, collar bones, and shoulders (small pause). Fill your arms, your wrists, and hands (small pause).

So many bones that help you carry and lift. Express who you are as you move, write, drive. Our bones give the structure that forms the shape of our bodies and the shapes of our lives. They hold the stories of our lives and our ancestors. "I know this to my bones," we find ourselves saying.

Your bone tissue has been with you since shortly after conception, forming a tube to protect your nervous system. Your bones truly hold the store of your whole life. (small pause)

Fill the bones of your face and skull with breath (small pause).

Feel your entire bone structure, your whole skeleton. So strong, wanting to support you, giving you the structure to move through the world. (small pause)

Now fill your bones with white light, breathe the white light deep into your bones, filling every space and breathing out any discomfort. Breathe in the light and breathe out that which doesn't feel good. Breathe in the light of healing and breathe out the stories that do not serve any more (small pause).

Light in, old stories out. Healing in, that which doesn't serve out. Keep breathing in light and letting go of the old as you breath out. Stay with the breathing in and out.

If something uncomfortable comes up, breathe it out, let it go into the stones and rocks around you, any thoughts and stories that you are holding on to breath them out and light in (about four minutes longer if you think they are okay with it. Every thirty seconds or so remind them to breathe. You will want to watch them, making sure no one is having to strong a reaction. Tears are fine; fear or terror is not).

Now take a breath and thank the rocks for receiving what you let go.

Bring yourself back to filling your bones with your breath. Ask your bones if there is a color of light they would like you to breath in: red, orange, green, purple... any color that will help your bones to feel stronger, healthy, and flexible (small pause).

Fill every joint with this color as you breathe in. Breathe in and feel the bones and joints in your feet fill up with the color. On your next breath, fill the bones in your calves, your knee, the femurs in your thighs (small pause).

Breathe in and fill your hips and your pelvis (small pause).

Now take a deep breath and feel each vertebrate and joint coming up your spine fill with this nourishing color (small pause).

Feel your rib bones and collar bones fill with color, your arms and wrists and hands. (small pause)

Breathe in and fill the bones in your neck with color; fill your face bones and skull (small pause).

Every bone in your body becoming healthier and stronger.

Take a deep breath and feel your whole skeleton alive and full of color.

Thank your bones for supporting you as best they can. Ask if there is anything they would like you to know in this moment. It can be a word, a symbol, a picture, maybe a feeling, even a new story (small pause).

Thank your bones for whatever you received, knowing that even if nothing perceptible came, you received something (small pause).

Now take a few breaths and start to feel the rest of your body, your muscles, your skin, your face. Take a breath and start to wiggle your toes and fingers.

As you bring yourself back to the space around you, when you are ready, staying quiet, pick up your journal and start to write. Specifically write your new story, what you are changing.

Summary: The rituals and meditations in this chapter are very powerful for releasing negative feelings, then finding and creating new stories to live by. They can be repeated periodically, but give at least a month in between the group rituals. The personal ritual using the bowl of water as your focal point is great to have going continuously. The meditations can be done more frequently.

Chapter 7

Vision

As we learned in Chapter 3, vision, purpose, and passion for life are really important to recovery and daily living. Sometimes as we heal, we simply want to know what to do next, or we need to understand our purpose in life at this moment, have something outside of ourselves that we can focus on for a while or long term that reignites us and helps us move forward though the process of recovery. Something that gives us something to dream about, to see what the other side of the process can look like when we are healed.

We also need to find what brings us hope and joy. A reason to go deep and look at our pain. Many people never recover fully because it is so painful to face our past so we can release it. At least if we can find some little things to bring us joy that are healthy for our being, we can make it through more easily. Know there is something we can go to.

It is also important to establish our connection to source, to god, to whatever our beliefs are. Finding this connection to source is so critical to our healing especially since many of us who have dealt with the trauma of abuse may have cut our connection to source/God or are very angry because we do not understand why we had to go through what we had to go through, especially as children, and so blame source/God. Reestablishing our connection can help us to find our passions and dreams, our visions.

We align with our inner light and heal deeply, regain our passions and visions, start to live our dreams without being pulled by the pain.

Rituals and Meditation

Dream and Vision Personal Altar

Because dreams and visions really need to be nurtured, creating a place (preferably in your bedroom) where you will see what represents them when you wake and before you sleep is really nice. Also as you take your clients through the rituals in this book, especially the ones where they create personal objects, this can be a place to put them.

The vision and dream altar is where you put objects that represent your visions and dreams. Right now, that may be as simple as a piece of paper with the word freedom or inner peace on it. It may be a picture or object that represents your fully healed self. Later, you can add items that represent your dreams for your future and take away the ones that have come true or are no longer relevant.

There is a personal ritual described after this one that, when done sitting in front of this altar, can help your client go even deeper.

Time: Ten minutes.

Purpose: Create the altar as a focal point to represent your dreams and aspirations for your future.

Materials: A place such as a table or shelf in your bedroom, cloth to cover, candles, objects that represent you and your healing, a journal to use as your dream journal

Steps:

1. Have your materials with you.
2. Invocation: Call on god, spirit, and your future self, as well as guides to help you to see clearly what is next, to

be able to visualize fun and joy in your future, to see yourself being healthy, strong, brave—whatever words bring you hope and comfort, peace, and knowing life is always growing, changing and becoming better. You are dedicating this space to this vision.

3. Cover the space with the cloth, then place the candle and items on the altar in a way that is pleasing to you. Over time, these items will change as you grow. You can add new ones and remove some. As you grow and your visions change, so will this altar.

4. Closing: There really is no closing to this altar. As you gain insights, thank spirit/god, your guides, whatever your belief system supports for those insights and visions.

Personal Ritual/Meditation: Daydream My Tomorrow

If your clients can do this once a day starting for five minutes and then moving up to fifteen, it can really help in the tougher times. Even a few times a week is good. They can do this as they go to sleep or when they first wake up. It will help them to sleep more easily and to wake up starting the day in a good place emotionally.

It is nice if you can walk them through this before they do it on their own. They will want their journal with them.

Time Needed: Five to fifteen minutes a day.

Purpose: Daydreaming, spending time to simply allow themselves to dream about their future. Science has shown that this actually reprograms the brain/mind and releases all kinds of feel-good chemicals when done with positive intent. It programs us to start thinking more positively.

Materials: Journal and pen, and a comfortable place to sit. They can do this in bed as they go to sleep.

Steps/Meditation:

If you are guiding them through, follow these steps. When on their own, they will freely flow.

1. Have them get comfortable whether sitting or lying down. Put their left hand on their chest and the right on the belly (like in the grounding cord ritual in Chapter 5). Take a few slow breaths in for three and out for five.

2. Have them imagine that they truly can do anything they want—paint beautiful pictures, build tree houses, ride a horse, scuba dive, dance, fly through the clouds. You know your clients well enough to fill in some things they might be attracted to at this time. They can daydream their perfect career, friendships, relationships. Anything that is positive and helps them to feel good.

3. And literally have them daydream about this just like they did when they were kids.

4. You can bring them to the now by asking what they would love to do most today. What would bring them joy? How about the future? Do they like what they do now for a living; if so, what would make it more enjoyable, more fun? What would their dream lifestyle be like?

5. Pause after each question to give them the time to daydream.

6. After a few minutes, have them write in their dream journal what happened in their daydream. Did they have any new ideas of something they may actually like to start? Did they remember something they really wanted to do like paint or dance but forgot about, places to see? Everything is alright; there is no right or wrong answer when it comes to daydreaming.

7. If they do this before going to sleep, when they first wake up, they can write what they discovered from their dreams or any insights they have as they wake in their journal.

As an Evening Ritual:

Once you get comfortable and are ready to sleep, ask your inner heart, your soul, to give you dreams that will help you, that will give you the answers you desire. You can ask a specific question or for insight around a particular situation. You can ask to integrate what you learned through the day or what is needed next in your journey. Writing this in your dream journal before you go to sleep can be helpful for looking at your dreams tomorrow.

Don't worry if you don't remember your dreams; we all dream, and insights come.

As a Morning Ritual:

I remember one of my teachers Sobonfu Somé saying, "When we wake up every morning, it is important to welcome ourselves from all the journeys we have taken while we were asleep. So, we wake up, we hold ourselves, and we welcome ourselves back."

When you wake, take a moment to hold yourself, to love yourself, to feel the warmth and life in your body. Your spirit and soul has been journeying in your dreams, and now it is home. After you welcome yourself back, ask what it is your soul brought back from your dream time. Make some notes in your dream journal. Know that your inner heart, the part of you that is so wise and truly has answers to all your questions, is there to guild and help you

Group Ritual

My Healed Self

Create an object that represents you when you are free again
Time Needed: If it's the full ritual, four hours; if only sharing time as a group, two hours. You can do the meditation in your

private session and have your client create the object before the group sharing session. Your set up time is about an hour depending on how much stuff you bring

Purpose: Create an object that represents your healed self. This is so powerful because it represents the future, where your client is going to. It is a reminder that there is an end to the pain. The project can be a drawing, a piece of jewelry, painted stones, decorating a doll, whatever medium you and your clients are comfortable working with.

This ritual can be done privately or in a group. The power of the group is each of your clients will feel heard, witnessed, and strengthened by hearing all the stories. As a group you will want to schedule four hours with them. You can do it as a mini workshop. You can also have your clients create this object on their own and then, in a group of shorter duration, present them to each other. It is also nice in conjunction with a releasing ritual, done after releasing ritual is completed.

Materials Needed: You will want to provide art materials and space to work like tables and chairs. Have this set up before you start the ritual. Ask your clients to bring items that are special to them, that bring joy and a sense of peace and recovery. They can incorporate these into their project. They can also bring their own materials to use and share if they choose.

Additionally, bring candles, cloths to decorate the altar, and pictures of themselves throughout their life in happy situations, also a journal and pen. You may want to have some scarfs available to cover their eyes if they are comfortable with this.

1. Clear the space with sage, incense or essential oils.

2. Once everyone arrives have each say their name and be welcomed by the group. Explain the purpose of this ritual in your words and the process for about five minutes. Meditate, create your object, and share it with the group. Remind them this is not who has created the best sacred item. Leave perfection and self-judgement outside! They will want their journals and a pen handy for the meditation. If they have already created their object, the purpose is to share their vision of their healed self.

3. Before you start the ritual, have your clients create the altar using the cloths, candles, pictures of themselves, and objects they brought or their completed object if this is the shorter ritual. Do not light the candles. If you like you can have the altar ready and they just place their pictures and objects on it.

4. Have chairs and/or space to lie down in front of the altar in a semi-circle, or if there is space have them build the altar in the center so they can be in a circle around

it. If you're only performing the sharing part, chairs and the altar are all the space that is needed

5. Open the sacred space. Call in their guides, god, angels, Jesus, whatever works for this group. Additionally, call in their future whole and joyful selves and their inner child to help them.

6. Guided Meditation: If this is the sharing-only ritual, skip this part.

7. Have everyone get comfortable facing the shrine, sitting or lying down with their journals and pen handy.

8. Have them take a moment to focus on their pictures and the objects they brought and the beauty they see there.

9. After a few moments, have them shut their eyes (If you can dim the lights, this is a good time to do that; if they want, they can use scarfs to block out the light if that is distracting to them).

Meditation Dialogue

Take in a few deep breaths. In and out, filling your lungs fully and really breathing out, letting go of everything not needed in this moment (small pause).

Now focus on your hearts, put your left hand over your heart and right hand on your belly. Take a few more breaths, feeling your heart, your center (small pause).

Now visualize you are sitting next to a fire. It can be a camp-fire, fireplace, bonfire, beautiful candle, whatever comes is perfect (small pause).

Really see it—the flames flickering, the colors. Can you hear fire wood crackling and popping or is it silent? Can you feel the warmth (small pause)?

This is your moment through the fire to connect with your future self. You may see your reflection in the fire or maybe feel a presence next to you. Let your future self be as tangible as possible (small pause).

Now ask your future self to give you a sense of what it feels like in the future when you are free and joyful (small pause).

Be trusting and kind to yourself (small pause).

Ask your future self if there is anything she wants you to know, a piece of advice you can use now (small pause).

Then ask: Is there a color, symbol, or word that is important for me at this moment in time (small pause)?

Is there anything else your future self wants you to know (small pause)?

Now feel your hands on your heart and belly and know that what your future self has told you will stay with you and is in your heart (small pause).

Over time, this knowledge will be added to and will grow (small pause).

Now thank your future self for all they have shared (small pause).

Take a few deep breaths, anchoring all you have seen, felt, and learned into your heart and body (small pause).

Take a deep breath in knowing that your future self is there to guide you and hold you as you come closer to her through time.

Now take a few deep breaths and start to sense the room, the sounds, and your body (small pause).

Wiggle your toes and fingers (small pause).

Stretch, and while remaining quiet, write in your journal about the meditation. If you like, get your pictures or objects and have them close while writing, go ahead and get them (If you dimed the lights, this is a good time to bring them up).

1. Creating future-self object: Two hours is recommended for this part of the ritual. After giving them time to write, have them go to the tables and start to create the sacred object of who they are in the future. Let them know how much time they will have and that if it doesn't get finished, they can do that later. Some may be resistant. You know your clients: Guide them; help them to at least get something started.

2. If they are doing this part on their own, you will have taken them through the meditation so remind them to

take a moment, maybe even read what they wrote in their journal, before starting the project on their own.

3. Sharing: Give each person time to share. Five minutes is a good timeframe. So if you have twelve people, you will need an hour for this. With a smaller group, you can give them more time to share or extend the time they have to work on their object.

4. Ask them to share what they believe their future self will feel like, be doing, etc.

5. Close the sacred space. Thank their guides, God, etc. for being present to help; thank their future selves and inner child for all they have done.

6. Post ritual: If they have created their dream altar, have them place what they create there. If not, ask them to place their future self somewhere where they will see it a number of times throughout their day, maybe even share what they learned with someone close and supportive, someone who can hold the vision with them without judgement.

Summary: Being able to see a future where we are healed and having a place to come to and renew these dreams and visions is so important when healing from abuse and trauma. The dream altar is the place where we can come daily to rejuvenate and know we have purpose in the world. By putting the objects there that represent our dreams and future, we can see ourselves more clearly.

Chapter 8

Honoring Ourselves

T his one is big. In the process of recovery, honoring the changes, the transformations, is so important. We have transformed and changed so many things—the way we think, the way we perceive others and ourselves. We've gone from victim to warrior, then to wise women strong in ourselves, speaking our truth and asking for what we want.

In indigenous cultures, there are many types of initiation ceremonies. For example, when children reach adolescence, there will be a ritual that incorporates the letting go of childhood and the moving into young adults. Then there's a ceremony when they become a woman or man after they have studied the ways of adults during their adolescence.

And just the same as when we are healing from abuse especially childhood, there is a need to honor our inner child, the little girl inside; hold her and thank her for showing up, and create rituals that honor her and allow her to come out, to play and have fun.

Another process of deep change we have gone through has included removing the "masks" we hide behind to become more honest so we can look deeply at ourselves. This doesn't mean we have gotten rid of all the masks. It is more about becoming aware of the ones that we used to hide from ourselves.

For example, I have my mask that I call charisma. This one is great when I need to deal with a large group of people I don't know well. I need to be charming, present and confident. Most of the time I feel this way, but if some insecurity comes in I can feel myself put on this mask which makes me feel more at ease and therefore I can be more open and honest with those around me and myself. Seeing when I use this on myself when I'm going to do something that my gut is saying no to was a big step in my growth.

In addition to realizing our masks, when we have learned to say yes to healthy changes, we need to have rituals to honor this. Having the courage to recognize when the environment we live in, whether mental or physical, is no longer healthy and making the change to what is right helps us deeply to gain confidence. Honoring this change is important.

This is where rituals and ceremonies are so helpful. For example, if you know a change is coming, you can do a releasing ceremony to let go of what is holding you back or simply to recognize it is time to let go of that which holds us and then perform a ceremony to celebrate your step forward.

Rituals and Meditation

Personal Ritual

This one is very simple yet can be a challenge at first.

Every night for thirty days, after you have brushed your teeth and gotten ready for bed, spend five minutes looking at yourself in a mirror. It needs to be big enough to see your whole face at least. If you have a full-length mirror you can stand in front of, that's even better.

While you gaze in the mirror, notice only the beauty and perfection.

At first, this can be really challenging, but you can always find something. Start with the color of your eyes, really looking deeply into them. Thank them for seeing the world around you. Next, notice your nose and honor it for bringing breath into your body.

Honor your ears for hearing and giving you the ability to listen. Honor your lips and mouth where you are learning to speak your truth. If you have a full-length mirror, honor your body for giving you a presence in this world, for mobility, for sensation.

Do your best not to see the flaws someone else told you that you have. If this were a sweet child in the mirror, you would say kind and loving words to her. You are a sweet child inside; be kind and loving to yourself.

Once you are finished, you can write in your journal for a few minutes how this process feels and how it feels different after you have done it a few times.

When you turn the lights out to sleep, tell yourself, "I love you, honor you and cherish you."

Ritual—Honoring Our Sacred Family with Masks

Masks are very powerful transforming and honoring tools. Just about every culture I know of uses them. They can represent gods, nature spirits, and ourselves.

You can create a mask that represents one of the behaviors in ourselves that we want to honor because it served us in the past, and now we are ready to release it: for example, playing the victim or putting on the "I am strong and don't need help" persona.

Make a mask of all-natural material to represents this. Then have a fire ceremony and burn it, sending it to rest with god. You can release the mask in a river where it can float away, dissolve, and be cleansed and purified by the water. You can place it in nature to dissolve into the earth. No matter what, always remember to thank the part of you it represents for how it served you.

I still have a mask I created many years ago. It represented my wanting to run away from challenges, even die at times, because I was so overwhelmed with sadness and grief. When I sit with it and think of what it meant when I created it, I realize how strong and resilient I am. It is a reminder that I can make it through anything. Because it was created in a group, it reminds me to ask for help, that I am not alone. I still learn something every time I sit with it, and it is a way of honoring myself.

Time Needed: Four hours minimum for ritual if creating one mask in a group, and an hour on each side for setup and cleanup. Making a full day or overnight is great for all three masks (explained in next paragraph); remember to provide meals or have them bring their own. It is easier than going out for lunch.

You can use this ritual to create masks to honor the different side of yourself. For example: one to honor your inner child, one for your maiden (some cultures call this the feminine), and one for your warrior (also known as the masculine). In a tradition I have learned a little of from Hawaii, they feel we have our own sacred inner family. When this is healthy in us, we are healthy with ourselves and the relations we have in the world. The masculine and warrior side is our father. The feminine or maiden is our mother, and our inner child is us.

Sometimes our warrior has become dominant keeping us "safe" in the world and needs the nurturing feminine. Sometimes, we have spent so much energy just getting through the day that we have forgotten that our inner child needs to play, to find joy and fun in the world. When we are in balance, these parts of our being all help each other instead of dominating one another.

This ritual is to create the masks that represent each of the aspects in the previous paragraph: inner child, maiden, and warrior. Men and women have these aspects. If this is a half day, you will realistically only have time for one. In this case, you will need to modify the meditation to have them find the one that wants to be created today. If you have a full day or overnight, all three can be made and honored. With the overnight, it can be really nice to include the earth mandala ritual where they create it before starting the ritual, then revisit it and change it after each mask.

Materials: Something to create the masks out of. This can be heavy paper that can be cut, premade plain masks, wooden masks—if you look up plain masks on Amazon or go to a local craft store, you can find different types. Have enough for everyone to have at least one (three if doing the longer ritual) and about fifty percent extra. We make mistakes!

Glue, glue gun, and tape.

Glitter, feathers, fabric, decorative stones, paint… All kinds of art supplies, or you can just have a few simple items. Whatever you have will work. I find that paper, cloth, and wooden masks work best for painting and some glues. You may want to experiment with the masks before the ritual. If you are not comfortable with crafts, find someone who is and ask them to join the ritual as an assistant.

Tables to work on and newspaper or cloth you don't care about to cover the tables. This is a messy process; it is for their inner child!

You may want the participants to bring items of their own to decorate with. I have a friend that would bring beads and beading supplies.

They will want a journal, and you can have paper and pens available if they forgot.

Candles, cloth, and flowers to put on the altar.

Ritual: Follow the basic structure laid out in Chapter 4.

Steps:

1. Clear the space with sage, incense or essential oils.
2. Create the space. You'll need a creative space where tables, chairs, and art supplies are located and a space for the altar where the blank masks are at the beginning of the ritual and where they will put their masks when finished to share. Have the space ready when they get there except maybe the altar if you want them to create it.

3. Once everyone has arrived, have each person say their name and the group welcome them. Then explain the purpose of the ritual and process. Have them build the alter if you have not.

4. Invocation. Because this is for them to get in touch with the three aspects of their self, make sure to call in their inner child, maiden and warrior to help them see them and find a way to represent them in the masks they create, as well as God, their guides, angels, whatever beliefs this group has.

5. After the invocation, have them pick out a mask from the altar and have it with them during the meditation. If they will create three masks, have them pick three.

6. Meditation

Items in () are for you to do, not part of what you will say while facilitating this meditation. Small and long pauses are relative to the time you have for the meditation and your clients ability to stay present with you. Too fast and they don't have time to process and do what you just said. Too long and they will be distracted.

Meditation Dialogue: For the One-Mask Ceremony

Get comfortable sitting or lying down with your journal, pen and mask next to you (small pause).

Take a deep breath in and let it out with a noise like a sigh, in again and out, really releasing anything outside this room from your mind. You are here to be with yourself, your inner child, your maiden, and your warrior (small pause).

Place your left hand on your heart and your right hand on your belly. Feel your breath as your body expands with the in breath and comes in with the out breath. Take a few nice slow breaths (small pause).

Now visualize you are out in nature, a field or meadow, a forest, by a river or the ocean maybe in the mountains (small pause).

See the beauty that is there. Are there grasses, flowers, trees (small pause)?

Boulders, water flowing (small pause)?

What does the sky look like? Is it clear? Are there clouds? Is it raining or snowing? (small pause)

Is it warm or cool (small pause)?

How does it smell (small pause)?

Is it night time, day time, sunrise, or sunset (small pause)?

As you are there enjoying this beautiful place, someone starts to walk toward you. You know in your heart they are kind and loving (small pause).

You notice their age, the way they are dressed, the color of their hair, their skin (small pause).

They come closer, and you are both standing or sitting together looking at one another, and you realize this is you, one of your inner selves, your maiden or warrior, your inner child (small pause).

Take a moment to notice how they look. Is there a scent to them? You are smiling at one another (small pause).

Take a moment to thank them for being with you, a part of you, and supporting you through your life (small pause).

Feel the love they have for you and you for them (small pause).

Ask if there is something special you can do in your daily life to honor them (small pause)?

Ask if there is anything special they would like on the mask you are creating to honor them, something to remind you of their love and support (small pause).

Take a few moments now to again feel their love and support, feeling it flow into your heart and belly through your hands, spreading throughout your body and filling you up with love and joy (small pause).

Know that this sense of peace and belonging is always available to you (small pause).

Now become aware of gravity supporting your body (small pause).

Become aware of your breath again and the room around you, knowing that the part of you that showed up is still there, always loving and supporting you and know you know them and can return the love and support, knowing they are always there for you to call on for guidance (small pause).

Take a few deep breaths and start to wiggle your toes and fingers becoming present to the room again. And when you are ready open your eyes, write about your experience, and when you are done, go and create your mask.

Meditation for the Three-Mask Ceremony

If this is a full day or overnight ritual, you will want to use this meditation and take three masks from the altar.

Get comfortable sitting or lying down with your journal, pen, and masks next to you.

Take a deep breath in and let it out with a noise like a sigh, in again and out really releasing anything outside this room from your mind. You are here to be with yourself, your inner child, your maiden, and your warrior.

Place your left hand on your heart and your right hand on your belly. Feel your breath as your body expands with the in breath and comes in with the out. Take a few nice slow breaths (small pause).

Now visualize you are out in nature, a field or meadow, a forest, by a river or the ocean, maybe in the mountains. See the beauty that is there. Are there grasses, flowers, trees (small pause)?

Boulders, water flowing (small pause)?

What does the sky look like? Is it clear? Are there clouds? Is it raining or snowing (small pause)?

Is it warm or cool (small pause)?

How does it smell (small pause)?

Is it night time, day time, sunrise, or sunset (small pause)?

As you are there enjoying this beautiful place, three people start to walk toward you. You know in your heart they are kind and loving (small pause).

You notice there is a little child, a woman, and a man (small pause).

You notice their ages; are they young, older? (small pause).

How are they dressed? What is the color of their hair and skin (small pause)?

They come closer, and you are standing or sitting together looking at one another, and you realize these amazing beings are you, your inner selves, your maiden and warrior, your inner child, your sacred family (small pause).

Take a moment to notice more deeply how they look. Is there a scent to them, an aura about them (small pause)?

You are smiling at one another (small pause).

Take a moment to thank them for being with you, the parts of you that are supporting you through your life (small pause).

Take a moment to feel the love they have for you and you for them (small pause).

Ask if there is something special you can do in your daily life to honor them (small pause).

Ask if there is anything special they would like on the masks you are creating to honor them (small pause), something to remind you of their love and support (small pause).

Take a few moments now to again feel their love and support, feeling it flow into your heart and belly through your hands, spreading throughout your body and filling you up with love and joy (small pause).

Know that this sense of peace and belonging is always available to you (small pause).

Now become aware of gravity supporting your body (small pause).

Become aware of your breath again and the room around you knowing that your inner child, maiden, and warrior are always loving and supporting you, and now you know them and can return the love and support, knowing they are always there for you to call on for guidance and to play with (small pause).

Take a few deep breaths and start to wiggle your toes and fingers, becoming present to the room again, and when you are ready open your eyes, write about your experience, and when you are done, go and create your mask.

1. Create the mask/masks. During this time, make sure they are working and staying relatively quiet and focused in a meditative state. Have food ready if they are there for lunch. If using the earth mandala ritual, remind them to go to their mandala in between each mask. For a shorter ritual, have snacks for them.

2. Share.

For the One-Mask Ceremony

After a couple of hours, whether they are finished or not, have them place their mask on and around the altar. You will want to gauge your time, so everyone has five minutes to share.

Ask them to share how the process was and what they learned to take away with them.

For the Three-Mask Ceremony

For the three-mask ritual, make sure there is a break for lunch. You may want to meet for a few minutes after lunch to get them focused if they had to go out or simply have them work on the masks through lunch making sure they brought a lunch and also have something for those who forgot! If it is an overnight retreat, have them meet at night, and you can do another ritual or meditation, maybe teach them the daydream ritual. Make sure when they do their sharing the next day, you give them ten minutes each to share about their masks: what the process was like for them, what they learned, how will they continue to honor their relationship with their sacred family.

1. Close the space. During the closing prayer, remember to thank their inner selves for being with them and loving them and creating a sacred link to themselves.

You know your clients and can help to make additional honoring ceremonies. For example, if you have started a group, when someone accomplishes something, you can take a moment in the group to honor them for what they accomplished and to support them in the next step. This can be as simple as recognizing them to the group and giving them a flower or a special card the group has signed. We do this for birthdays; why not for times when they have made a major move forward, like leaving a relationship that has not been good for them or standing up for themselves against a family member?

Honoring ourselves is so important to healing. The daily ritual of teaching your client to honor their body can help them to start seeing the beautiful person they are. Having their masks that represent their feminine, masculine, and child on their dream altar gives them a chance to see their internal landscape and keep it balanced.

Chapter 9

Obstacles You May Encounter

When I started to write this chapter, I thought, "There are no obstacles to using ritual!" Then I realized that for the most part that is true in my life today, but I have been using rituals for many purposes for so long that they truly are part of my everyday life. So, I took some time to take a look at myself years ago.

One of my biggest obstacles when I was starting to participate in rituals was that I expected instant results! Some of this was because I did feel such great difference the first time I was involved in a releasing ritual; I thought they should all be that way.

I was too inexperienced to realize that some of the rituals I didn't feel were that great were actually very powerful. When I look back at them now, I can see how they affected me long-term and opened the door to deep change.

In the West, we have been trained to want instant results, big bangs of insight, and to be healed right away. Our clients can especially feel this way when the magnitude of what they have taken on sinks in. The difference is most insight and healing from ritual continue to unfold over time. If we stay connected to how the ritual made us feel, to our dreams and meditations afterward and to our thoughts after the ritual is over, we can continue to grow, change, and heal. Many times, small or subtle changes have the most profound effect.

Another obstacle was finding the time. When I really started wanting to use ritual, I was married, had a child, was teaching in the computer industry and traveling two weeks out of a month, seeing clients, owned a farm, and Lord knows what else. How was I going to fit this in?

The first thing I did was find a mentor who could help me. Then I started to do little rituals a couple of times a month. I started a women's group that met once a month, then started going on weekend retreats a few times a year. I set aside time to just be with my daughter—this became a ritual I did not want to break! Ritual helped me to start to see what was really important in life.

For most of us, time and confidence are probably your biggest challenge to moving forward adding these practices into your practice. If you are like most of us, you run on a pretty busy schedule and fitting something new in to learn can feel complicated.

As a therapist, you can incorporate small rituals into your sessions with your clients. With just two or three of you, say in couples' therapy, you can easily do a short and sweet ritual around vision or letting go and bringing in something new. You can meet once a month with a small group at your office.

Eventually, you will know exactly how you want to use ritual and ceremony with your clients. A really nice thing is a ceremony when your clients have a breakthrough. It can be as simple as giving them a pretty stone to help them remember the moment. You can even get some of the pens from a craft store for decorating stones and have them write a word or symbol on the stone to remind them of the break through.

Because ritual is so powerful, without knowing it, the part of our subconscious mind that wants us safe, wants to avoid change, and most of all that wants to be accepted, can stand in our way. It can put obstacles in our way and bring up our own fears and doubts. You might find yourself thinking, "I don't know enough. I can never do this. My clients will think I've gone nuts."

After years of practicing ritual and ceremony, I still have some form of doubt and fear come up. I try to simply thank my mind for wanting to keep me safe and move on.

Sometimes clients can be resistant to introducing new methods into their therapy. Change can be hard. When I come back from a teaching or weekend retreat, I will often say, "I just learned something new. Will you try this with me? I think you will like it."

For a person new to this, I may do a simple guided meditation and have them hold a stone during the meditation and ask them to keep the stone with them to remind them of what they felt during the meditation or to carry a stone with them and when the have a bad moment visualize it going into the stone. The next time they see you, have them throw away the stone, put it back in nature whether on the ground or in a river or stream. These are some simple ways to introduce them to ritual. Many people have heard of worry stones.

I know quite a few therapists and counselors who have clients who love the incorporation of these practices and those who don't. The nice thing is ritual is another tool you have in your pocket to help. Use ritual with those who are open, and stay with traditional therapy when that is what the client works best with.

Another interesting challenge is having preconceived notions or expectations. I have gone into rituals just knowing that a certain person was going to have really great results, finally release the attachment to a memory really troubling them, find forgiveness for themselves, or get an answer to a question.

The ritual starts, finishes, and they didn't feel anything big or ended up with a different insight than I thought they should have, or whatever I thought should happen didn't. We cannot control ritual; we want to let it flow. Some are really good at that. I had to learn it! I can be a bit of a control freak.

Once I started to trust the process and let the ritual evolve organically out of the structures I had learned, amazing transformations started to happen, and everyone got what they need even if it may not be what they or I wanted for themselves

Ritual is about flow within structure. When we finally let go of the control and learn to flow, ritual becomes part of us.

Once the structure is learned, you will get a feel for the flow and become comfortable with the elements of the ritual and their meaning, and create your own.

Finding the time to immerse into each element and understand its meaning, its essence, and then to feel confident leading others in ritual is wonderful.

There is enough information in this book to start. Working with each section for a few weeks and feeling it yourself will help you gain confidence. Maybe introduce it to your clients through the guided meditation or even go to a workshop to have someone guide you through the process.

There are always challenges when learning a new technique or process. The first is simply becoming familiar so that you gain competence which in turn gives you confidence. As you gain more confidence, you will feel more competence. It's the getting started part that can distract us.

It took the dedication of Sobonfu, my other teachers, and myself over time for me to become comfortable and easy with ritual, and it has taken the support of my closest friends and colleagues to grow.

Chapter 10

Conclusion

My hope for you, dear reader, is that after reading this little book you have some understanding of the importance ritual and ceremony can be in helping your clients heal. Having traveled that path of healing, I know what a difference it made for me. I also know what a difference it has made for hundreds of people who want to feel whole, stop the emotional pain, and be free.

The reason I wrote this book was to provide a tool, a process that can be used by you to help your clients move through their emotional pain more quickly and easily, and to help you help your clients toward freedom.

Ritual and ceremony can become a part of the tools your clients and you can use throughout life to both celebrate and heal when life challenges come up.

For example, when my mother died, I started to use the water altar we discussed in Chapter 6. Having the bowl of water there helped me to have a focus for my grief to go to and for me to release in the morning to the earth.

Chapter 4 gave you an understanding of how ritual has been used for centuries and helps at deep levels in the psyche to bypassing the mind and help the subconscious release the beliefs that hold us back. Chapter 4 also gives you the overview and the step by step procedures for facilitating rituals, for creating small groups and for retreats around ritual where you can take your clients deep and help them feel really supported, and even to create a community that learns more rituals and does them together once a month.

I believe once you become comfortable and incorporate these tools into your life and practice, you will appreciate their value.

There are plenty of rituals to get you started on your way with your clients in Chapters 5-8. These chapters talked about each type of ritual particularly suited to healing from abuse, yet they can be used in many circumstances to support transformation and healing.

And you have learned to tailor ritual to your client's needs and traditions and beliefs.

As I look back over the writing of the book, I realized two things: one, how much I always want my clients to have as many tools available to heal as possible, and now I want others to have these tools also; and two, when I started sharing rituals with others, how much I changed and grew.

For those of us who are dedicated to helping others, I think there is no greater joy than witnessing the transformation from pain to joy and freedom and seeing people who have lost their center find it and become grounded and strong in their lives again.

Please email, heidi@delightinlife.com and let me know your thoughts and how I can help. I am available for individual and group training.

Ritual and Ceremony Check List

1. Materials List
2. Setup
   a. Clear Space
   b. Create alter
   c. Set up seating
   d. Set up work space
5. Welcoming ritual
6. Explain purpose
7. Invocation
8. Ritual

9. Closing
10. Give any post instructions
11. Follow up with the clients in one week

Bibliography

John Bradshaw, *Healing the Shame that Binds You.* (HCI; October 15, 2005).

John Bradshaw, *Homecoming: Reclaiming and Championing Your Inner Child.* (London: Bantam; February 1, 1992).

Joe Dispenza, *Evolve Your Brain: The Science of Changing Your Mind.* (HCI; January 15, 2007).

Bruce H. Lipton, *The Biology of Belief: Unleashing the Power of Consciousness, Matter & Miracles.* (Authors Pub Corp; March 18, 2005).

Dr. Matt James, *Ho'oponopono: Your Path to True Forgiveness.* (Carlsbad: Crescendo Publishing, LLC; October 6, 2017).

Carl Jung, *Modern Man In Search of a Soul.* (San Diego: Harcourt Brace; August 4, 1955).

C.G. Jung, *Psychology of the Unconscious.* (Dover Publications; January 27, 2003).

Dalai Lama, *The Universe in a Single Atom: The Convergence of Science and Spirituality.* (Harmony; September 12, 2006).

Sobonfu Some, *The Spirit of Intimacy: Ancient African Teachings in the Ways of Relationships.* (New York: William Morrow Paperbacks; January 5, 2000).

Sobonfu Some, *Welcoming Spirit Home: Ancient African Teachings to Celebrate Children and Community.* (Novato: New World Library; September 1, 1999).

Sobonfu Somé, *Women's Wisdom from the Heart of Africa.* (Sounds True; April 11, 2014).

Sobonfu E. Some, *Falling Out of Grace: Meditations on Loss, Healing and Wisdom.* (North Bay Books; August 1, 2003).

Acknowledgments

Where to begin? I have been so blessed to have so many amazing teachers, collogues, and dear friends along this journey called life. I remember times when I didn't even want to be alive, but through their kindness, generosity, insights, and love, I made it through very dark times.

With my teachers and friends pushing me and challenging me to go beyond my limits, I learned healing and wholeness is not just a possibility; it is a reality we can embrace. I wish there was room to name you all.

I want to thank Roselyn Breyer for teaching me that one of the main duties our family is here for is to create the "sacred wound" when we are children that will be our greatest teacher and challenge through life. Because of this, I can see the great wisdom and joy that was made possible in my life as I healed from this wound. Knowing about the sacred wound also allowed me to forgive those that I felt hurt me.

Additionally, it was through Roselyn that I met Mary Branch. Mary Branch has spent so many hours helping me move through my darkest times. Knowing when I needed to talk, use ritual or simple cry and be loved. Her confidence in me has been more then I could ever ask for. Her dedication to teaching and helping people heal is unconditional.

I especially want to thank Sobonfu Some' with all my heart for her deep, deep dedication to bringing the teachings of the Dagara to the west. Though I have studied multiple teachings, it is through her I found my real home inside. I miss her dearly, yet she is always here. I can feel her laugh, I feel her confidence in me and most of all her love. She taught me the importance of community, joy, and feeling our grief and pain. That we all are a gift to each other and we each deserve to be loved and cherished no matter what we may think of ourselves or feel we may have not done "right." She truly brought ritual and ceremony alive in a way I had never experienced before and in a way that healed my deep and hidden wounds. The Dagara are a gift to the Earth and because of Sobonfu we can know them.

Additionally, I want to thank my dear friend Susan Hough who is so dedicated to keeping the teachings of the Dagara alive as well as the people by raising money and putting wells into the Villages. Her voice is heard in many places. She is a gift.

And most of all, I want to thank to my amazing daughter Carrissa. She has always been my motivation to break the negative patterns of my childhood and ancestry, so she could live a full and joyful life. I am truly blessed that she chose me to be her mom.

Thank you to the Morgan James Publishing Team: David Hancock, CEO & Founder; my Author Relations Manager, Margo Toulouse; and special thanks to Jim Howard, Bethany Marshall, and Nickcole Watkins.

About the Author

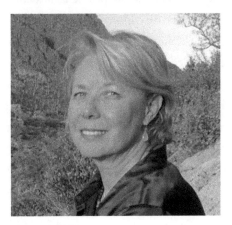

Heidi started her Journey at age seventeen, when she came across her first Indian yoga master who piqued her natural curiosity about the body and mind. From that point on, Heidi has been fascinated with how the world we live in and create for ourselves affects us and our well-being. She received her first certifications in applied kinesiology when she was twenty-one and has continued to study healing and the art of ritual and ceremony. Even while in corporate America teaching internationally in the computer industry, she continued to study internationally and work with clients privately. Finally, in 2001 after 9/11, she left her corporate position of twenty-five years, realizing her heart was in helping people to heal and feel whole.

When Heidi was fifty-four, all her childhood memories came flooding back, and it was not good. However, because of her extensive knowledge of ritual and ceremony, a counselor also very familiar with using Ceremony and Ritual and the community of friends she had to help her, she deeply and quickly healed, she felt whole and full within six months not the normal two to five years.

Heidi is so grateful to have studied with many wonderful teachers like Roselyn Breyer, Hyemeyohsts Storm, Debra Ray, and Sobonfu Some'. She has had the joy of spending time in the Peruvian Andes and Rainforest, Bolivia, Mexico, Europe, Nepal, and the United States, studying with the indigenous people.

In addition, she is a certified and licensed massage therapist, movement teacher, and health coach. She currently resides bi-coastally in Laguna Beach California and Northern Virginia spending time with clients, family, building a retreat center and enjoying life.

Thank You

Thank you so much for reading *The Guide to Using Ritual and Ceremony to Delight in Life!* If you're ready to continue your journey feel free to reach out to me at www.delightinlife.com.

There are additional resources on the website for you to use including guided mediation and written material. I'd like to hear from you and help you to learn more about ritual and ceremony.

May everyone you connect with feel your heart,
Heidi

CPSIA information can be obtained
at www.ICGtesting.com
Printed in the USA
LVHW042027120820
662929LV00002B/309

9 781642 798753